UNDERSTANDING FITNESS

Recent Titles in
The Praeger Series on Contemporary Health and Living

A Guide to Getting the Best Health Care for Your Child
Roy Benaroch, M.D.

Defending and Parenting Children Who Learn Differently: Lessons from
Edison's Mother
Scott Teel

Fact and Fiction of Healthy Vision: Eye Care for Adults and Children
Clyde K. Kitchen, M.D.

Ordinary Miracles: Learning from Breast Cancer Survivors
S. David Nathanson, M.D.

Solving Health and Behavioral Problems from Birth through Preschool:
A Parent's Guide
Roy Benaroch, M.D.

Polio Voices: An Oral History from the American Polio Epidemics and Worldwide
Eradication Efforts
Julie Silver, M.D. and Daniel Wilson, Ph.D.

When the Diagnosis Is Multiple Sclerosis: Help, Hope, and Insights from an Affected
Physician
Kym E. Orsetti Furney, M.D.

UNDERSTANDING FITNESS

How Exercise Fuels Health and Fights Disease

EDITED BY
JULIE K. SILVER, M.D., AND
CHRISTOPHER MORIN

The Praeger Series on Contemporary Health and Living

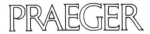

Westport, Connecticut
London

Library of Congress Cataloging-in-Publication Data

Understanding fitness : how exercise fuels health and fights disease / edited by
Julie K. Silver and Christopher Morin.
    p. cm. — (The Praeger series on contemporary health and living, ISSN 1932–8079)
   Includes bibliographical references and index.
   ISBN 978–0–275–99494–5 (alk. paper)
   1. Physical fitness. 2. Exercise—Health aspects. I. Silver, J. K. (Julie K.), 1965– II. Morin,
Christopher, 1964–
   RA781.U53 2008
  613.7′1—dc22   2008000237

British Library Cataloguing in Publication Data is available.

Library of Congress Catalog Card Number: 2008000237
ISBN: 978–0–275–99494–5
ISSN: 1932–8079

First published in 2008

Praeger Publishers, 88 Post Road West, Westport, CT 06881
An imprint of Greenwood Publishing Group, Inc.
www.praeger.com

Printed in the United States of America

The paper used in this book complies with the
Permanent Paper Standard issued by the National
Information Standards Organization (Z39.48–1984).

10 9 8 7 6 5 4 3 2 1

This book is for general information only. No book can ever substitute for the judgment of a
medical professional. If you have worries or concerns, contact your doctor.

Some of the names and details of individuals discussed in this book have been changed to protect
the patients' identities. Some of the stories may be composites of patient interactions created for
illustrative purposes.

We dedicate this book to our families, who have supported us throughout our careers and who understand the importance of exercise in health and disease.

CONTENTS

Contents

SERIES FOREWORD

Over the past hundred years, there have been incredible medical break-throughs that have prevented or cured illness in billions of people and helped many more improve their health while living with chronic conditions. A few of the most important twentieth-century discoveries include antibiotics, organ transplants, and vaccines. The twenty-first century has already heralded important new treatments including such things as a vaccine to prevent human papillomavirus from infecting and potentially leading to cervical cancer in women. Polio is on the verge of being eradicated worldwide, making it only the second infectious disease behind smallpox to ever be erased as a human health threat.

In this series, experts from many disciplines share with readers important and updated medical knowledge. All aspects of health are considered including subjects that are disease-specific and preventive medical care. Disseminating this information will help individuals to improve their health as well as researchers to determine where there are gaps in our current knowledge and policy-makers to assess the most pressing needs in health care.

Series Editor Julie Silver, M.D.
Assistant Professor
Harvard Medical School
Department of Physical Medicine and Rehabilitation

Preface

The scientific and medical communities agree that exercise, especially cardio-vascular, is of critical importance for the prevention and treatment of many diseases. However, there is quite a bit of confusion about what kinds of exercise are most important as well as how best to do them and at what intensity.

In *Understanding Fitness* we asked experts to write about what the research shows with respect to exercise. This is an "evidence-based" book for the intelligent reader who wants scientific answers to questions about how we move affects health and disease. Too often it is fitness gurus, who have never read a single exercise study, who offer advice to the public. This leads to misinformation and significant confusion. The media, too, is flooded with exercise information—some of it quite credible and some of it pure nonsense. How do you know the difference? Read *Understanding Fitness* and you'll be able to sort it out in the future.

Before you begin, however, it's important to clarify the terms "physical activity" and "exercise" as they pertain to this text. Often people use these terms interchangeably, but in research studies they are typically not synonyms. Instead, physical activity encompasses all human movement, most notably activities of daily living, while exercise is defined as planned physical activity with the goal of increasing fitness.

As you read it is likely that the research the experts cite will confirm much of what you already know. However, get ready for some surprises—there are many exercise myths that even health conscious individuals often don't realize are false. In *Understanding Fitness* you will get the most up-to-date information about exercise in health and disease. Hopefully that knowledge will lead to a healthier life for you.

Acknowledgments

We are grateful to the many people who helped make this book possible. First and foremost we want to thank the authors who contributed chapters to this guide. Their expertise and hard work is seen in every page. Debbie Carvalko is the extremely capable and energetic editor of the project who assisted us throughout the publishing process. Mary Alice Hanford coordinated the project and helped with the research and manuscript preparation. Jennifer Morin lent her expertise in exercise physiology as well.

1

HISTORICAL EXERCISE TRADITIONS FROM A HEALTH PERSPECTIVE

James Whorton

The last few decades have witnessed such a deluge of research demonstrating the health benefits of regular exercise that one might readily suppose the connection of physical activity to bodily well-being is a modern discovery. In fact, exercise has been recognized as a component of healthful living since Greek antiquity, at least, and has been pressed upon the public as a much-neglected responsibility for a full two centuries. To be clearly understood, then, our present preoccupation with strenuous activity should be viewed against the background of ideas and practices that have undergone steady evolution since the eighteenth-century Enlightenment. In examining that background, I will give attention to European origins, but from the early 1800s on will concentrate on developments in the United States. As will be seen, historical attitudes toward exercise and health have been shaped not just by medical science, but also by ideas and methods formulated by lay health reformers.

Western medicine traces its roots to the fourth-century BC Greek physician Hippocrates, who was the first writer to consistently interpret health and disease as conditions determined wholly by natural, rather than supernatural, agencies. Hippocrates placed heavy emphasis on the prevention of illness, recognizing that the surest way to remain healthy was to live in accord with the body's own natural mechanisms of functioning. The habits that were conducive to optimal functioning, furthermore, were easily discovered by experience: it did not take many late nights of rich food and strong drink to make most people realize that the path to feeling well lay elsewhere.

That path came to be known as "hygiene," a term derived from the Greek word for health and embracing all the activities relating to health over which a person had control. During the last 150 years, the meaning of hygiene has been narrowed to apply simply to cleanliness, but for most of Western history it referred to all the rules of behavior by which a person could ensure full vitality. For simplicity's sake, the rules were sorted into six categories during the second century AD, and eventually came to be identified in English literature as air, food and drink, sleep and watch, motion and rest, evacuation and repletion, and passions of the mind (emotional equanimity, stress management, if you will). While "air" was a qualitative category (one should seek air that is pure, free of smoke, dust, and foul odors), the others were quantitative, the observance of a Goldilocks ideal of just the right amount. Thus a person could eat pretty much whatever appealed to him or her (there were no basic food groups beyond breakfast, lunch, and dinner) as long as he or she did not gorge or starve himself or herself. Likewise, one should sleep neither too much nor too little, should avoid both diarrhea and constipation (evacuation and repletion), and should be neither manic nor depressed. "Moderation in all things" was the golden rule of hygiene.[1]

Motion and rest was the category for physical activity and moderation prevailed there as well. A certain amount of exercise was necessary to keep muscles and organs running smoothly, but periods of idleness were also needed to avoid deterioration from overuse. Through most of history, the standard for moderate exercise was one that strikes us today as falling well short of what is needed for serious physical conditioning. Daily walks were advised, not ten-kilometer runs, and activities such as dancing and singing were also recommended for cardiovascular fitness. But before dismissing the hygienists of old as lax and undemanding, it should be remembered that they were writing for people who moved about on foot or rode horseback, who tilled fields and otherwise used their bodies much more than is required of most people in modern urban society.

THE INDUSTRIAL REVOLUTION AND FITNESS

It was the Industrial Revolution of the late eighteenth century and the consequent shift from a primarily agrarian to a predominantly urban mode of life that brought forth appeals for more strenuous efforts at exercise. As it became apparent that the city would be the environment of the future, with sedentary employments in shops and factories the rule, hygienists began to despair. By the end of the 1700s, it was virtually obligatory for volumes on health to open with a chapter bemoaning the debilitating effects of "civilization" by contrasting life in the traditional village with that in the emerging metropolis. Time and again, the poor city dweller was dragged forth to have his stature measured against that of the farmer (and invariably to the former's humiliation). "Compare," physicians jeered, "the whistling plough-boy with the calculating stockbroker; the shepherd on the mountains with the merchant in the city," the "florid complexion and sound health of the country youth" with that of the "sickly sallow . . . city child." The country youth flourished almost by necessity, his vocation actually forcing him to partake of pure air, simple diet, regular hours, and, most of all, laborious daily exercise.[2]

But once philosophers of health got over the shock of the urban revolution, they realized that while the old days on the farm were gone, that did not mean that city folk were doomed to decrepitude. In the new age, people could still make a conscious effort to live by nature's rules of hygiene. Health would not come automatically, it would have to be pursued, but it could nevertheless be attained: "We no longer find health in our daily pursuits as a matter of course," an English hygienist explained; "the enormous growth of our towns, and the new set of evils contingent upon that growth have obliged us to set to work to find counteracting agencies." There, in a nutshell, was the history of health promotion since 1800, a history of the elaboration of regimens of exercise and systems of diet that allow one to live naturally in an unnatural environment.[3]

In the nineteenth century, the medical profession played only a limited role in encouraging the pursuit of health. Faced with a host of lethal infectious diseases that annually caused a much greater percentage of the population to die than is the case today, physicians focused their attention on treatment rather than prevention. To the extent that they did address health maintenance, they offered the same old advice on exercise. More ambitious programs of health promotion did attract individual medical practitioners, but such men (and later in the century a few women) were generally regarded by colleagues as eccentrics, at best. Nevertheless, it was from such seemingly fringe programs that a preventive consciousness that stressed the value of exercise took form.

GRAHAMISM AND MUSCULAR CHRISTIANITY

The ideas that prevention was far superior to cure, that health was a positive state of exuberant vitality and not mere absence of disease, and that human life could be significantly lengthened by cultivating a natural lifestyle even while immersed in the artificial existence of modern civilization were the creations of a populist health reform movement that began in the 1830s under the name of Grahamism. The nominal leader of the movement, Sylvester Graham, was a Presbyterian minister turned antialcohol crusader who then expanded his outlook on health to denounce all unnatural appetites, not just Demon Rum. Meat-eating, he believed, was one of the most injurious things a person could do to himself: the Graham cracker was America's first health food, created as the cornerstone of the vegetarian diet he was the first to promote for reasons of physical and not only moral health. Just as harmful, if not worse, was sexual activity outside marriage and in excess of the frequency required for procreation (once a month was the maximum safe rate of venery and that only for the still young and robust); Graham was the primary instigator of the Victorian notion that sex is not just bad, but bad for you as well. So restrictive an allowance for sexual indulgence might suggest that Grahamites did not believe in physical exertion, but in fact strenuous exercise was strongly encouraged. Running was recommended over walking, for example, though for no greater distance than a mile or so. Singing, on the other hand, was to be done only in church, not at parties, and dancing was frowned upon under any circumstances.[4]

Grahamism, also known as the popular health reform movement, was concentrated in the northeastern states and attracted only a few thousand serious adherents. As might be apparent, it advocated a system of physiology that was dictated by morality, and physical health was important ultimately as a stage in the construction of an ideal Christian society. In this, it was paralleled by another movement that emerged later in the century, "muscular Christianity." But while Grahamism advocated exercise as one part of a broad program that embraced diet, dress, and other elements of hygiene, muscular Christianity focused on exertion alone. First voiced in the 1850s in the novels of Englishmen Thomas Hughes (*Tom Brown's Schooldays*) and Charles Kingsley, this philosophy contended that robust physical power was not incompatible with the gentle morality of Christian teaching, but, on the contrary, was essential for the performance of God's (and the nation's) work. Muscular Christianity had a profound cultural impact, elevating the building of strength and endurance to the level of spiritual duties and promoting athletic competition in particular as an essential tool for building Christian character. By the end of the 1860s, it was a public article of faith that "he who neglects his body . . . commits a sin against the Giver of the body. . . . Round shoulders and narrow chests are states of criminality," muscular Christians sermonized; "it is as truly a man's moral duty to have . . . strong arms, and stalwart legs, . . . as it is to read his Bible or say his prayers."[5]

The author of the foregoing homily on health also proposed that "there would be more godliness in this land, and more manliness, too" if half of the nation's churches were converted to gymnasiums. He was here pointing to a specific program of exercises that had taken the country by storm since the early 1860s, the "New Gymnastics" of Dioclesian Lewis. There was an old gymnastics, the German system of exercises similar to today's Olympic gymnastic events. But while German *Turnen* had been brought to the United States in the 1820s, it had caught on only with young and daring males. Dio (his preferred name) Lewis, a former physician, saw the need for workouts that could be managed by both sexes and all ages, exhibiting particular concern for improving the health of women through his new gymnastic activities. A few female authors had previously tried to persuade women to engage in regular calisthenics (most notably Catharine Beecher, sister of Harriet Beecher Stowe), but with much less success than Lewis. It was his system, incorporating dozens of stretching, bending, and throwing exercises involving wooden dumbbells, beanbags (that he invented), hoops, wands, and other devices, that first stimulated large-scale female participation in programmed exercise; like aerobics classes that would flourish in the following century, the exercises were often performed to the accompaniment of music. Lewis was also the pioneer in America in the training of instructors of exercise classes through the Normal Institute for Physical Training he founded and operated in the 1860s and 1870s; in line with his goal of elevating women's health, he set the tuition of female students one-third lower than that of male pupils.[6]

The Lewis system was quickly adopted in schools throughout the country. It was not, however, calculated to make Christians or anyone else all that muscular. It aimed at creating flexibility and coordination (and for the ladies, beauty and grace) along with strength, but to develop real brawn one had to turn to a competing exercise program of the 1860s, the strength-building regimen of George Windship. The next-to-smallest student in his Harvard class, Windship was the role model for the folkloric weakling who gets sand kicked in his face: when the class bully threw his books down a flight of stairs, young George took up weightlifting and returned some weeks later to face his tormentor down. But Windship did not stop there. After matriculating at Harvard Medical School, he undertook the invention of weight machines that in basic design were identical to many of the pieces of equipment found in weight-training rooms today. By 1861, the 5-foot 7-inch, 143-pound "Roxbury Hercules" was astounding audiences by dead-lifting several times his body weight. Preceding his demonstrations of might with lectures on the theme "Strength Is Health," Windship set off a "lifting mania": "Like mushrooms after rain," a contemporary marveled, "lifting machines sprang up in parlors and offices and schools everywhere."[7]

SARGENT'S SYSTEM

One of those caught up in the lifting mania was a teenager named Dudley Allen Sargent, who, much as Dio Lewis had done with gymnastics, would democratize weight-training, making it more accessible to the general population. Sargent earned a medical degree from Yale, then in 1879 took the position of professor of physical training at Harvard. Recognizing that strenuous lifting was not to everyone's taste and ability, he developed the Sargent System of training structured around exercises on pulley-weight machines (many of his own invention) that could be adjusted to the strength of the individual and directed toward the cultivation of specific muscle groups. Sargent's System proved so attractive that by the end of the century it was being employed to some degree in 250 colleges, 300 public school systems, and 500 YMCA gymnasia.[8]

Sargent's System was at the core of a new professional discipline of physical education that spread through colleges and schools in the 1880s and 1890s. Professors of physical education, moreover, were for the most part physicians; the medical profession was at last taking the lead in developing more ambitious exercise programs. Students nevertheless were too often unimpressed, finding the repetitive lifting and calisthenic drills prescribed for them boring. Physical educators soon came to realize that if the same ends could be achieved by means that were more spontaneous and enjoyable, more people would participate, and do so with more energy. Thus the promotion of exercise for health transformed in the late 1800s, passing from "the gymnastic era" of rigid exercise routines to "the athletic era" of participation in competitive sports. Rowing, running, and rugby, already revered for their efficacy in training muscular Christians, were joined by baseball, football, and cycling as forms of exercise that were suitable for broad-scale participation because they were as enjoyable as they were strengthening. Thus by 1900, the basic forms of physical conditioning popular today—calisthenics, weight-training, and sports—were firmly in place.

As people—the younger ones, at least—took up athletics in unprecedented numbers, though, many physicians began to experience second thoughts: might not the excitement of athletic striving drive some participants beyond the golden rule of moderation and lead to injury? Armed with only the most rudimentary knowledge of the long-term effects of repeated exertion of the muscular system, heart, and lungs, it was only natural for physicians to err on the side of safety and fear danger where a later, more sophisticated generation would see invigoration. By the opening of the twentieth century, a medical backlash was forming against athleticism, a reaction that posited a range of supposed debilitating effects from overindulgence in sport and vigorous exercise.

THE ATHLETE'S HEART

One concern dominated all others in the discussion: "athlete's heart." Some of the readers of this chapter no doubt are of an age to remember being warned away from running and other physical activities because of the risk of developing athlete's heart, an enlarged and enfeebled organ that augured premature death. Some enlargement of the heart muscle does indeed result from strenuous exercise, but it is a normal response to training that represents an improvement in cardiac function. Many doctors, however, believed this physiological hypertrophy to be pathological, essentially the same as the cardiac dilatation associated with heart disease. First rowing was condemned as a heart destroyer, then long distance cycling, then distance running. The last brought on the direst warnings of athletic suicide when the revival of the Olympic Games in 1896 sparked something of a craze for the marathon (the Boston Marathon was initiated the following year). Yet when all was said and run, statistical studies of longevity of marathoners, cyclists, and rowers revealed they actually lived to more advanced years on average than nonathletes. By the 1910s, progressive medical thought regarded the athletic heart as the ideal, an organ strengthened by regular physical exertion, rather than damaged. It nevertheless took two decades for the profession as a whole to accept that view and one can only guess at the number of athletic careers needlessly ended, the amount of pleasurable and healthful recreation forbidden to people throughout their lives, and the degree of hypochondria and anxiety suffered by athlete's heart "patients."[9]

Early twentieth-century discussions of athlete's heart and athletics for health are revealing also for signaling a change in the cultural rationale for exercise. The religious underpinnings of nineteenth-century discourse had hardly disappeared; sport was still seen as a moral enterprise, particularly as a builder of character. But when expounding on the ultimate goals of exercise, writers were much less given to citing personal holiness that would bring in a Christian utopia. American society had changed. The explosion of industrial productivity and growth of economic prosperity following the Civil War had fostered a mindset more attentive to the satisfactions of the present world. The qualities bred by athletics—strength, stamina, perseverance—now appealed primarily because they could be seen as aids to success in the world of business. The pursuit of health was in the long run the pursuit of wealth; physical expenditure brought fiscal rewards.

The gospel of prosperity as preached in the early 1900s praised one attribute above all: efficiency, the elimination of waste in time, effort, and money. Physical educators of the day took the cue, promoting physical efficiency as the most desirable result of exercise. The athlete's heart, for example, was superior because it pumped blood and oxygenated muscles more efficiently than the untrained organ. Physical efficiency was also, however, intimately tied to diet. Indeed, the discipline of sports nutrition, an integral component of physical training today, has its roots in turn-of-the-century enthusiasm for improving the efficiency of body machinery by determining the ideal materials with which to build and maintain the machine.

Enthusiasm is not too strong a word to describe the excitement felt by physicians and biochemists at the beginning of the twentieth century over the revolutionary discoveries being made in the science of human nutrition. For most of history, diet was supposed to be quite a simple, purely quantitative matter: you could eat what you wanted as long as you didn't eat too much of it (or too little). It was recognized that physical activity increased dietary needs—pugilists had to eat more than professors—but the only qualitative dietary distinction made for athletes was the recommendation of large quantities of meat. Competitors were presumed to benefit from flesh food because the fiercest animals were carnivores.

EVOLVING BIOCHEMISTRY

As biochemistry began to emerge in the early 1800s, it became possible to chemically analyze foodstuffs, so that by 1840 fats, carbohydrates, and proteins had been determined to be the three main groupings of dietary compounds. The physiological role that each group played, however, was not clarified until the end of the nineteenth century. By that time, the dietary importance of various minerals was being experimentally demonstrated as well, and during the first two decades of the twentieth century the nature of vitamins would be clarified. There was thus ample justification for scientists of the day to hail the dawning of the age of "the newer nutrition," as they called it, a nutritional science that represented a quantum leap beyond the nutritional knowledge of the past.[10]

With respect to exercise, the chief impact of the newer nutrition was to encourage the consumption of more carbohydrate and less protein. Authoritative texts at the start of the century were still recommending as much as 150 grams of protein a day for athletes, a ratio of grams of protein to kilograms of body weight several times higher than what is advised today. That figure was a holdover from the nineteenth-century assumption that since muscle tissue was composed of protein, the energy for muscular exertion must come from oxidation of protein: the more one exercised, the more protein one needed. The newer nutrition, however, recognized that the energy for muscular activity was derived from the combustion of carbohydrate, not protein, and so exercise did not require a high-protein diet. That was the new theory, but old beliefs die hard and the protein myth proved particularly tenacious, being dispelled only by the example of one of the most extraordinary physical specimens of American history.

Horace Fletcher was a *bon vivant* whose love of food led to a crisis of obesity in middle age, which he was able to overcome only by adopting the practice of thoroughly chewing every bite of food until it was reduced to pulp before swallowing. As a rule, the practice demanded a hundred or more chews per bite, and so through the combination of time, tedium, and jaw fatigue, Fletcher came to eat much less food and to lose most of his excess weight. He never regained the athletic build of his youth, remaining somewhat portly, but he did achieve an astonishing level of muscular endurance. In his late forties, after years of physical inactivity, he decided on a whim to go bicycling and ended up pedaling more than 100 miles—without fatigue and without muscular soreness the next day. He attributed the feat to the purification of his body through thorough mastication, supposing his food was divided so minutely that it was all absorbed into the body, leaving nothing behind to form intestinal waste that could decompose and poison the system (Fletcher boasted he had bowel movements only every few weeks and the matter voided was both small in amount and odorless). His claims of exceptional endurance because of elevated physiological efficiency brought him to the attention of the professor of physical education at Yale, who had him undergo a battery of physical tests (sit-ups, knee bends, etc.) designed for members of the Yale rowing team. Fletcher surpassed the undergraduate record in every test, both the first time he performed, in 1902, at age 54, and the second time, four years later.[11]

How Fletcher did what he did remains a physiological puzzle, but at the time it seemed even more amazing because he did it on a much lower protein intake than was believed necessary. His demonstration so surprised Russell Chittenden, the Yale professor of biochemistry, that he took the lead in calling for reevaluation of the dietary protein recommendation, resulting in the much lower level accepted as the standard today.

Fletcher's example also gave heart to vegetarians, who since the days of Graham had believed their diet was best for health but had never convincingly demonstrated it. Now inspired by evidence that high-protein food—meat—was not essential for athletic achievement, vegetarians in Europe and America dedicated themselves to winning as many athletic competitions as they could so as to prove beyond question the superiority of their diet. This "muscular vegetarianism," as it might be called, resulted in a number of impressive victories in distance walking, running, cycling (led by the aptly named Englishman James

Parsley), even tug-of-war, and vegetarian literature continues to the present to tout athletic success as evidence of the healthfulness of the diet.[12]

The debates over exercise and nutrition, and exercise and cardiac health, are indicative of the intrusion of science into evaluations of the benefits of physical activity in the early twentieth century. Physicians and physiologists alike began to subject exercise to experimental study in an attempt to determine the biochemical and physiological mechanisms of exertion and identify the specific benefits, risks, and optimal levels and limits of strenuous exercise. In the United States, the most notable investigations were conducted at the Harvard Fatigue Laboratory, established in 1927, where trailblazers in sports medicine demonstrated, among other things, that endurance exercises actually did strengthen the heart and enhance "the efficiency of the human body as a machine."[13]

POORLY CONDITIONED AMERICANS

In the meantime, despite physiologists' and physical educators' best intentions, many Americans were neglecting physical conditioning. The problem was dramatized most powerfully by the rejection of hundreds of thousands of young men from military service in World Wars I and II because they could not pass the physical examinations required for induction; in the Second World War especially, the physical strength of the population was thought of as a matter of national security. Then, in 1953, a widely publicized survey of muscular fitness among American schoolchildren discovered that more than half "failed to meet even a minimum standard required for health," while fewer than 10 percent of European children scored that low. These findings were startling and sparked a reaction akin to the public response to the Sputnik launching four years later; the fitness gap demanded national attention and remediation every bit as much as the science gap. President Eisenhower himself directed attention to the problem, eventually convening (in 1956) a President's Conference on Physical Fitness, which led to the creation of the President's Council on Youth Fitness, a body of athletic notables that recommended requiring more physical activity in the schools and the adoption of periodic tests to measure the fitness of schoolchildren. The American Association of Health, Physical Education, and Recreation soon designed a set of seven physical achievement tests to be administered to students in grades five through twelve, which was ultimately adopted by forty-three states. In 1963, President Kennedy, aiming to improve health at all ages, renamed the government body the President's Council on Physical Fitness; under the further revised title of the President's Council on Physical Fitness and Sports, it is still active in promoting exercise.[14]

The postwar concern to elevate Americans' levels of fitness was reflected as well in the founding of a new medical organization: The American College of Sports Medicine (ACSM). Established in 1955, the ACSM drew together physicians, physiologists, physical educators, and other professionals committed to the promotion of exercise for health. In the half-century since its establishment, the college has been a pacesetter in encouraging research in exercise physiology, publishing journals to educate professionals in the science of fitness and the public in the principles of healthful living, developing programs for training and certifying fitness instructors and personal trainers, devising exercise testing formats to measure levels of fitness, and prescribing exercise regimens to aid the unfit and rehabilitate victims of cardiac and other ailments.[15]

As in the nineteenth century, public awareness of the benefits of exercise has also been stimulated over the last 100 years by individual lay health reformers. Chief among these during the first half of the 1900s was Bernarr Macfadden. Born in 1868 to an alcoholic father and tuberculous mother, Macfadden was orphaned before his teenage years and plagued by weakness and illness throughout adolescence. He fought back with dumbbells and distance-walking, gradually building himself into a man capable of teaching gymnastics classes and winning professional wrestling matches. By 1899, Macfadden had formulated a program of gymnastic exercises and weight-lifting that he dubbed "Physical Culture," the science of cultivating a body both beautiful and brimming with strength and energy. *Physical Culture* magazine also appeared in 1899 and quickly became the leading source of popular instruction on exercise and health into the mid-1900s. Macfadden was a prolific author of books as well, among these were *Vitality Supreme, The Power and Beauty of Superb Womanhood,* and *The Virile Powers of Superb Manhood.* This last book expressed a distinctive characteristic of the physical culture approach to health. The polar opposite of the prudish Sylvester Graham, Macfadden (who reveled in posing all-but-nude for the camera and audiences) believed that sexual exertion was the most invigorating of all forms of exercise, and his second wife testified that he was dedicated to practicing what he preached. He also preached that the practice of physical culture equipped one to succeed in the business world and demonstrated that principle as well through his Physical Culture Publishing Company, one of the largest publishing empires in the country, one that specialized not just in health literature, but in true crime and (of course) true romance magazines. Finally, he practiced the longevity he promised as a reward of physical culture, living to the age of 87 (despite his habit, adopted in his eighties, of parachuting from an airplane every birthday).[16]

Macfadden's system embodied two main exercise emphases—the stimulation of physical efficiency and the sculpting of a muscular body as palpable evidence of that efficiency. In that second objective he was joined by several other advocates of what would come to be called bodybuilding in the 1940s. One was Angelo Siciliano, anointed by Macfadden in 1922 as "America's Most Perfectly Developed Man." Assuming the name Charles Atlas, he marketed a system of "dynamic tension," a set of isometric exercises that he swore had transformed him from "a 97-pound weakling" into a magnificent physical specimen. But more significant for the rise of bodybuilding both as a health-promoting activity and as a competitive sport were Bob Hoffman, of York, Pennsylvania, and Joe and Ben Wieder, brothers from Montreal. From the Depression years onward, all were active in manufacturing and marketing barbells, in publishing bodybuilding magazines, and in organizing bodybuilding competitions (the chief institution in the sport, the International Federation of Bodybuilders, was founded by the Wieders in 1946 and now has member organizations in 175 countries). In 1978, Joe Wieder established the National Strength and Conditioning Association (NSCA), which has grown into an organization with nearly 30,000 members in more than fifty nations. NSCA is dedicated to disseminating "the most advanced information regarding strength training and conditioning" in an effort to encourage greater and more effective participation in weight training. Wieder has also followed the example of Macfadden in building a major publishing company dedicated to promoting health through exercise: *Muscle and Fitness* and *Shape* are two of the most popular health magazines in the United States.[17]

THE IMPACT OF THE MEDIA ON FITNESS

Meanwhile, physical conditioning without the use of heavy weights had also grown into a mass participation activity, thanks in large part to the development of new media that allowed instruction to be extended to a wider audience. The first to successfully exploit the power of television to stimulate people to exercise in their homes was Jack La Lanne ("the Godfather of Fitness," he has been called), whose exercise show aired as early as 1951. La Lanne is now in his nineties and still going strong as an internationally renowned champion of the strenuous life. During the 1970s, workout videos began to be utilized, most notably by Richard Simmons and, the following decade, Jane Fonda, who famously pushed devotees to exert themselves to the point of making their muscles "feel the burn."[18]

While many used such videos in the privacy of their homes, others decided they could be motivated to greater effort exercising in company. As in the late 1800s, gyms began to proliferate in the 1970s, expanding from small independent exercise clubs into international chains such as Gold's Gym, which began as a bodybuilding emporium in Muscle Beach (Venice, California) in 1963, and today is the largest coeducational gym chain in the world. Gold's more than 600 outlets, furthermore, have stretched services far beyond the original concentration on weight training to the provision of treadmills, rowing machines, and other exercise equipment, and, as new programs have evolved, to Pilates training, spinning, and more—even kickboxing. A still more remarkable venture has been Curves, a gym catering specifically to women. Opening its first facility as recently as 1992, Curves is now the largest fitness business in the world, boasting 10,000 locations worldwide.[19]

The manufacture of weight machines, treadmills, and numerous other forms of exercise equipment has become a major industry in response not just to the needs of fitness clubs, but also to soaring demand for in-home use. Yet the most notable version of physical conditioning outside the gymnasium to emerge over the past half-century is one that requires no more sophisticated apparatus than sturdy shoes. Jogging and running (the distinction between the two is a matter of pace) have drawn adherents since the mid-nineteenth century. But as the mass-participation activity so familiar to us all today, it dates to the late 1960s. In 1966, Bill Bowerman, track coach at the University of Oregon, published a short book titled *Jogging* that sold several hundred thousand copies and set off unprecedented enthusiasm for the activity (the following decade Bowerman would cofound Nike, the running shoe company that heralded a new era of specialized footwear for amateur joggers; Bowerman also developed the waffle design for running shoe soles). In 1968, Texas physician Kenneth Cooper authored *Aerobics* (a word he coined), which became a bestseller and Book-of-the-Month Club selection. At once an appeal to Americans to become more active for the sake of health and an easy-to-follow guide to ways of accomplishing that goal, *Aerobics* rated different types of exercise on their effectiveness in improving cardiac and respiratory function. On that basis, Cooper constructed a system of points earned for each activity according to time and level of intensity and encouraged people to strive for certain weekly point totals as a measure of aerobic benefit and progress toward improved condition. Although a variety of physical activities was included in the system (swimming, cycling, walking, jogging, even running-in-place), running was put forward as the most valuable. Cooper has continued as a leader in exercise promotion through the Cooper Institute in Dallas, where clients enroll in a Wellness Program that blends aerobic exercise and weight training with diet and stress management (www.cooperinst.org). Further, like the ACSM, Institute staff also conduct research in exercise physiology and supervise educational programs to certify several thousand students a year as physical trainers for health clubs and gymnasia (much as Dio Lewis did at his institute in the mid-1800s).[20]

The next great stimulus to the jogging boom was Frank Shorter, a distance runner from Yale who in 1972 became the first American since Johnnie Hayes (1908) to win the Olympic marathon. Shorter's victory at the Munich games riveted national attention on the marathon and motivated thousands to take up distance training in pursuit of the goal of completing a marathon. Registration at the Boston Marathon, the premier event in the sport, graphically illustrates the explosion of interest in the grueling race. In 1964, the race drew barely 400 entrants; in 1984, the figure was nearly 7,000. In 2007, more than 20,000 completed the race. The New York City Marathon now has to run a lottery to select its more than 30,000 entrants from twice that number of applicants.[21]

In the decade following Shorter's gold medal, the marathon took on mythic proportions as a test of both conditioning and character. Where in the early 1900s physicians worried that participation in a marathon could destroy an athlete's heart, in the mid-1970s, some physicians asserted that distance running was so beneficial that anyone completing the marathon in less than four hours would make himself/herself immune to heart disease. The race was also embraced as the ultimate test of determination and ability to withstand pain, being made, in effect, into a philosophy of life. Another bestseller, George Sheehan's *Running and Being*, presented distance running as the path to self-discovery, inner peace, and confrontation with human mortality, a kind of muscular existentialism for the secular modern world.[22]

In 1976, Frank Shorter placed second in the Olympic marathon in Montreal, further solidifying Americans' interest in the event. The following year, another American runner, James Fixx, published a volume—*The Complete Book of Running*—that shot to the top of the *New York Times's* nonfiction bestseller list and stayed there for more than a year. The book appealed in great part because it presented running and jogging not from the perspective of an Olympic-caliber athlete but from that of an average person who had been an overweight smoker who then slimmed down and broke his addiction through running. But in 1984, at the age of 52, Fixx died of a massive heart attack during his daily run, stirring up anew fears that running was a danger to cardiac health. As it turned out, there was a history of heart disease in his family (his father had died of a heart attack at the age of 42) and ultimately the moral most people drew from his death was that his life had likely been prolonged by running.[23]

CHANGING PATTERNS OF DISEASE

Broader public participation in exercise activities has been further encouraged over the last several decades by changing patterns of illness. For most of human history, the chief threat to health and most frequent cause of death was infectious disease. As recently as the nineteenth century, life expectancy was kept below 40 by the prevalence of such ailments as tuberculosis (the leading cause of death throughout the 1800s), typhus, cholera, yellow fever, diphtheria, and a swarm of other germ-caused illnesses. With the development of microbiology during the last quarter of the century, however, not only were the agents of infection identified, but it became possible to disrupt the routes of transmission of infectious organisms and thus prevent their spread. The subsequent decline in mortality from infection resulted in a sharp increase in life expectancy: in the United States, average longevity rose from 47 in 1900 to 71 in 1970.[24]

But as the population grew older, degenerative diseases associated with aging (heart disease, stroke, cancers, diabetes, and others) became much more common. In 1900, heart disease was responsible for only 8 percent of deaths in the United States; by 1960, 40 percent of deaths were due to heart disease. By that time, however, research was accumulating to demonstrate that chronic, degenerative ailments could be prevented to some degree by lifestyle changes, particularly through smoking cessation, proper diet, and exercise. In 1979, in fact, a *Surgeon General's Report on Health Promotion and Disease Prevention* called for the mounting of a second public health revolution to follow the revolution in reducing infectious disease, a campaign to attack the "new killers and cripplers," chronic diseases. Increased physical activity was proposed as an important component of that campaign. The latest *Surgeon General's Report on*

Health Promotion and Disease Prevention, published in 2001, places "Physical Activity and Fitness" at the very top of its list of twenty-two "priority areas" for improving the nation's health.[25]

Yet while distance running continues to draw hordes of participants down to the present, rates of obesity among Americans have risen dramatically over the past three decades. Television, computer games, soft drinks, and fast food have conspired with other socio-cultural forces, not least trends in public schools that allot less time to recess and physical education, to breed a population in greater need of bodily exertion than perhaps any in history. Government studies following up the 1979 *Surgeon General's Report* have been uniformly discouraging with respect to the public's attention to exercise. One found, for example, that in 1990 the recommended goal of twenty minutes of strenuous activity at least three times a week was being met by only 5 percent of Americans. Nearly two decades later, *Newsweek* reports (in 2007) that "only 31.3 percent of people age 18 and older in the United States engage in *any* regular leisure-time physical activity" (emphasis mine). Despite the efforts of Lewis and Sargent and Cooper, eighteenth-century warnings of the erosive effects of urban, industrial civilization seem more apt than ever.[26]

However, for the hundreds of thousands who do regularly exercise, whether at home, in the gym, or on the road, there is much satisfaction in the mounting research findings that support the value of physical exertion for bodily and mental health and for longevity (a particularly striking demonstration of the benefit of exercise came from the Cooper Institute in 1989, with the publication of a study demonstrating a direct correlation between low levels of physical fitness and risk of death from all causes). Today's physically active legions might well join voices with their counterparts from an earlier time in singing an anthem composed by the valedictorian of the 1863 class of Dio Lewis's Normal Institute of Physical Training, "The Song of the Gymnasts":

Now, gymnasts strong, lift we high a song
For our art and its triumphs glorious,
That leads the van for the health of man,
And is over ills victorious![27]

NOTES

1. Jack Berryman, "The Tradition of the 'Six Things Non-natural': Exercise and Medicine from Hippocrates through Ante-bellum America," *Exercise and Sport Sciences Review*, 17 (1989): 515–559.

2. Thomas Trotter, *A View of the Nervous Temperament* (Troy, NY: Wright, Goodenow and Stockwell, 1808): 89–90; James Johnson, *The Influence of Civic Life, Sedentary Habits, and Intellectual Refinement on Human Health and Human Happiness* (Philadelphia, PA: Hope, 1820): 47.

3. B. R. P., "The Ladies Sanitary Association," *The English Woman's Journal*, 3 (1859): 74.

4. James Whorton, *Crusaders for Fitness: The History of American Health Reformers* (Princeton, NJ: Princeton University Press, 1982): 3131.

5. Moses Tyler, *The Brawnville Papers* (Boston, MA: Fields, Osgood, 1869): 162–163; Bruce Haley, *The Healthy Body and Victorian Culture* (Cambridge, MA: Harvard University Press, 1978).

6. Jan Todd, *Physical Culture and the Body Beautiful* (Macon, GA: Mercer University Press, 1998).

7. George Windship, "Autobiographical Sketches of a Strength-seeker," *Atlantic Monthly*, 9 (1867): 102–115; Dudley Sargent, *An Autobiography* (Philadelphia, PA: Lea and Febinger, 1927): 98.

8. Dudley Sargent, *An Autobiography.*

9. James Whorton, "Athlete's Heart: The Medical Debate over Athleticism, 1870–1920," *Journal of Sport History*, 9 (1982): 30–52.

10. Elmer McCollum, *A History of Nutrition* (Boston, MA: Houghton Mifflin, 1957).

11. James Whorton, "'Physiologic Optimism': Horace Fletcher and Hygienic Ideology in Progressive America," *Bulletin of the History of Medicine*, 55 (1981): 59–87.

12. James Whorton, "Muscular Vegetarianism: The Debate over Diet and Athletic Performance in the Progressive Era," *Journal of Sport History*, 8 (1981): 58–75.

13. Jack Berryman, "Historical Background, Terminology, Evolution of Recommendations, and Measurement," in *Physical Activity and Health: A Report of the Surgeon General* (Atlanta, GA: U.S. Department of Health and Human Services, 1996): 19; Jack Berryman, *Out of Many, One. A History of the American College of Sports Medicine* (Champaign, IL: Human Kinetics, 1995): 11.

14. C. W. Hackensmith, *History of Physical Education* (New York: Harper and Row, 1966): 466–474, 494–496; Hans Kraus and Ruth Hirschland, "Muscular Fitness and Health," *Journal of Health, Physical Education, and Recreation*, 24 (December 1953): 17–19; Deobold Van Dalen and Bruce Bennet, *A World History of Physical Education*, 2nd ed. (Englewood Cliffs, NJ: Prentice-Hall, 1971): 521, 545.

15. Berryman, *Out of Many, One*, www.acsm.org.

16. Whorton, *Crusaders for Fitness*, 296–304.

17. Robert Ernst, *Weakness Is a Crime: The Life of Bernarr Macfadden* (Syracuse, NY: Syracuse University Press, 1991): 114; Joe Weider and Ben Weider, *Brothers of Iron* (Champaign, IL: Sports Publishing, 2006).

18. www.jacklalanne.com; www.richardsimmons.com; www.jane-fonda.net.

19. www.goldsgym.com; www.curves.com.

20. Kenny Moore, *Bowerman and the Men of Oregon* (Emmaus, PA: Rodale, 2006); Kenneth Cooper, *Aerobics* (New York: Bantam, 1968).

21. Mary Carmichael, "Let's Get Physical," *Newsweek*, May 14, 2007, 62–66; www.bostonmarathon.org; www.runningusa.org; www.nycmarathon.org.

22. Thomas Bassler, "Marathon Running and Immunity to Heart Disease," *The Physician and Sports Medicine*, 3 (April 1975): 77–80; George Sheehan, *Running and Being. The Total Experience* (New York: Simon and Schuster, 1978).

23. Jane Gross, "James F. Fixx Dies Jogging," *New York Times*, July 22, 1984, 24.

24. Gerald Grob, *The Deadly Truth: A History of Disease in America* (Cambridge, MA: Harvard University Press, 2002); www.cdc.gov/nchs/fastats/lifeexpectancy.htm.

25. Gary Shannon and Gerald Pyle, *Disease and Medical Care in the United States* (New York: MacMillan, 1993): 45; U.S. Department of Health, Education, and Welfare, *Healthy People: The Surgeon General's Report on Health Promotion and Disease Prevention*

(Washington, DC: U.S. Government Printing Office, 1979): vii–ix; National Center for Health Statistics, *Healthy People 2000. Final Review. National Health Promotion and Disease Prevention Objectives* (Washington, DC: U.S. Government Printing Office, 2001): 65–69.

26. Andrea Piani and Charlotte Schoenborn, *Health Promotion and Disease Prevention United States, 1990* (Washington, DC: U.S. Government Printing Office, 1993): 8; Michael Miller, "Going From Fat to Fit," *Newsweek*, March 26, 2007, 50.

27. Steven Blair, S. N. Blair, H. W. Kohl III, R. S. Paffenbarger Jr., D. G. Clark, K. H. Cooper, and L. W. Gibbons, "Physical Fitness and All-cause Mortality: A prospective study of healthy men and women," *JAMA*, 262 (1989): 2395–2401; Thomas Higginson, "The Health of Our Girls," *Atlantic Monthly*, 9 (1862): 722–731.

2

CARDIOVASCULAR HEALTH BENEFITS

Matthew N. Bartels

Although modern medical advances and public health measures have allowed a much longer and healthier life for most people, the conveniences of modern life have also created the singularly unique problem of inactivity. The greatest current risk to reversing the improvement in mortality achieved in the last century is the many detrimental effects of physical inactivity and the complications of subsequent obesity. The multiple-faceted metabolic syndrome is characterized by a clustering of central obesity, insulin resistance, dyslipidemia, and hypertension. All of these are significant cardiac risk factors and the simple truth is that all of these can be ameliorated or reversed by exercise.

Since we will be discussing the benefits of exercise in the prevention and treatment of cardiovascular disease, a definition is needed to make clear what that actually encompasses. Cardiovascular disease includes heart disease, peripheral vascular disease, and stroke all under one umbrella. At first glance it may seem that this is a random grouping of disorders, but actually, they all share a common patho-physiological pathway: atherosclerosis of the blood vessels. Individuals with a stroke often have claudication (insufficient circulation to the legs) and individuals who suffered a heart attack are at greater risk of stroke and peripheral vascular disease. These diseases all have a common pathway, and fortunately, have a common preventative and restorative treatment—physical activity and exercise.

The cardiovascular benefits of exercise are an essential part of cardiac risk factor modifications and assist in the control of diabetes, improvement of blood pressure management, and improved lipid control. Exercise intervention is part of the standard recommendations for individuals with stroke,[1] coronary artery disease,[2] and peripheral vascular disease.[3] Still, an individual does not have to be a part of a formal program to be able to achieve these benefits. Even a moderate increase in daily activity will improve cardiovascular status and the modification of cardiovascular risk factors will garner benefits in the prevention of other disease, such as the prevention of renal failure, improvement in bone health, decreased pulmonary disease, improved sense of well-being, and improved immune function. Unfortunately, many individuals only modify lifestyle and incorporate good cardiovascular health habits after the onset of disease. It is primary prevention before the first event that it is essential for cardiovascular disease prevention. Lifestyle modification, which includes exercise, is an essential part of the prevention and treatment of cardiovascular disease that is within the control of the individual.

PREVALENCE AND INCIDENCE OF CARDIAC DISEASE

Despite the attention given to many other medical conditions, cardiovascular disease is still the most common cause of death and disability in the United States. Some startling statistics regarding cardiovascular health in the United States can be gleaned from the CDC reports on health behaviors of adults. The picture on leisure time physical activity is very alarming and is an area that most people can make a significant impact on their health. In the 2002–2004 time period, 38 percent of adults never engaged in any light moderate, or vigorous physical activity, with only one in eight adults engaging in any vigorous activity at least five times a week.[4] Additionally, women and older people performed less activity, and lower educational status and socioeconomic status were less likely to engage in physical activity. In the area of body weight, the nation has had a progressive increase in weight over the last fifty years, and in the most recent data, this trend continues.[5] Overall, nearly six out of ten adults were overweight or obese in the 2002–2004 survey and 23 percent of adults were obese. Overweight status was most common in adults between the ages of 45–74 years of age, being much lower for adults over 75 and under 45. Again, higher education was associated with a better health status; less obesity was associated with greater education. With regard to smoking, just over a fifth of all American adults were smokers.[6] Cigarette smoking also was associated with starting at a younger age—four in five smokers started smoking before the age of 21. Fortunately, more than 40 percent of smokers have tried to stop smoking in the past year. This trial rate shows that the message of the importance of smoking cessation or reduction is being heard by the general population.

Because of the lack of activity and obesity, cardiovascular disease is a leading health care issue in the United States. Fortunately, exercise is an important and effective part of the solution to the problems discussed and can have profound public health benefits. As an illustration, hospital discharges for people over the age of 65 show an incidence of 767.9/10,000 for heart disease, 175.6/10,000 for cerebrovascular disease, while all cancers combined account for 172.2/10,000 population.[7] The savings from even a small reduction in these numbers would be astounding, not to mention that the individual patients would be saved from illness and pain. Reviewing these numbers should provide a serious motivation to individuals to improve their own health status with a program of vigorous exercise as a part of a cardiovascularly healthy lifestyle.

OVERVIEW OF BENEFITS OF EXERCISE IN CARDIOVASCULAR DISEASE

In many ways, exercise can be thought of as the elixir of life since it has multiple benefits. Even modest exercise can achieve the goal of improved quality of life and decreased incidence of disease. The benefits fall into two broad categories, those that directly prevent disease or the recurrence of disease and those that cause a modification of other risk factors for cardiovascular disease.[1-4]

One of the direct benefits of exercise is found in the improvement of cardiac function. The heart is a muscle and with exercise it can improve in strength and endurance. One way that cardiac function is measured is by looking at cardiac output, a method describing how much blood the heart can pump. The goal is to improve efficiency of the heart as a pump and decrease the work it has to perform at any level of activity. Two separate components of heart function create the overall effect of cardiac output—one is the stroke volume (how much blood each beat of the heart can push out) and other is the heart rate. Thus the amount of blood pumped is described by a simple equation:

$$\text{Cardiac Output (CO)} = \text{Heart Rate (HR)} \times \text{Stroke Volume (SV)}.$$

Since the greatest strain is placed on the heart when it is going very fast, it is better to increase the pumping of the heart by improving the stroke volume. With exercise, the heart can significantly increase, even double, the amount of blood pumped with each beat.[8] This can lead to a resting heart rate that is now much lower than the preexercise heart rate. Since the maximum heart rate is relatively fixed (like the maximum RPM on your car engine), having a lower resting heart rate means that there is more reserve for exertion and that there is less strain at any given level of work (lower heart rate for any given load). This increase in efficiency means less wear and tear on the heart and a lower risk of cardiac disease. Similarly, when an individual exercises, the blood vessels also show an improvement in function.[9,10] These benefits are essential as a decrease in the stiffness of the blood vessels will allow the heart to work less, allow for better peripheral circulation, and lead to a lower incidence of stroke or peripheral vascular disease. The exact mechanisms by which exercise improves vascular stiffness are still being elucidated, but there are clear benefits.

The indirect benefits of exercise on cardiovascular disease by modification of other risk factors include improving diabetic control,[11] lowering blood pressure,[11] and lowering weight.[1-4] The nice feature of exercise is that the improvement in all of these risk factors can be achieved without costly medications or side effects. It is only the individual's effort that needs to be expended.

The most important indirect risk factor improvement with exercise is the maintenance of ideal body weight. Much has been made of the "epidemic" of obesity, and it is evident that there is a clear increase in the incidence of obesity. A great deal of research is being done to find the genetic and other causes of obesity and individuals, government, and other sources have spent billions of dollars in seeking improvements through diet and other weight loss schemes. However, the simple truth is that individuals are exercising less (including a generalized decrease in overall activity) and eating more. Another harsh truth is that effective weight loss is not achievable without a combination of diet modification and exercise. Weight loss involves a total change in lifestyle and that is the only way to sustain any weight reduction that may have been achieved. If one simply diets, the body turns down basal metabolism. With sufficient caloric restriction, one will eventually lose weight. But the diet is only a temporary thing, as soon as the target weight is achieved and the individuals go back to their previous eating patterns, then the weight will be regained as the body's set point was not changed. This is the basic reason dieters yo-yo between their target weight and their higher weight. With the addition of exercise and dietary modification—changing bad eating habits—the basal metabolism is maintained at a high level, and when a target weight is achieved, there is no see-saw as the individual is now living the right lifestyle to maintain their weight. The difficult part of this approach is that it involves a commitment to regular exercise; the benefit is that it works.

Additionally, diabetes control is essential. Fortunately, exercise can improve diabetic control, preventing many end organ injuries, including lowering stroke and peripheral vascular disease, decreasing cardiac disease, and preventing renal failure, neuropathy, and eye disease. As an added bonus in an individual with diabetes and ideal weight, exercise will reduce insulin resistance and will further improve sugar control. This will help to decrease the need for insulin injections or oral medications, but more importantly, will slow the development of atherosclerotic disease. Moderate exercise with walking or cycling will often be sufficient to achieve these benefits and can be built into a healthy and active lifestyle.

For healthy adults, the current American College of Sports Medicine (ACSM) guidelines recommend that individuals should exercise for twenty to sixty minutes three to five days a week in order to decrease cardiovascular risk.[12] Of all the exercises available, walking is the most convenient, cost effective, and easiest to perform. In Europe, walking is the most commonly used form of activity.[13–17] There are physiological and psychological benefits that have been well described.[1–4] Exercise improves health overall and improves cognitive and psychological function, but more importantly for this discussion of cardiovascular effects of exercise, improves cardiac function, reduces vascular stiffness,[18] and prevents stroke.[19]

Recent studies have shown some interesting findings regarding exercise and cardiovascular benefit. The benefit of exercise can be likened to that of a medication—as long as you take it and at an appropriate level, you get a benefit.[20,21] If you stop exercising, you lose the benefit, just as if you cease a medication, the benefit ends. In postmenopausal women, cardiovascular risk is increased by a rise in atherogenesis (an arterial disease characterized by the hardening and thickening of the blood vessels) due to a combination of increased blood pressure, worsened lipid profile, and increased obesity, especially central obesity.[20,21] The current accepted recommendation is thirty minutes a day of moderate intensity activity such as brisk walking every day of the week.[2] The best way to achieve this is to build exercise into one's daily routine. Unfortunately, trying to set aside extra time or getting up earlier to exercise will usually fail as people settle back into old habits. The location and timing of where exercise is performed is also important. By placing a treadmill in front of a television, an individual can combine exercise and a favorite daily program. Planning to exercise with a partner and turning exercise into a social event may also help, as it makes exercise more fun.

Benefits of Exercise in Peripheral Vascular Disease

Peripheral vascular disease (PVD) is a condition where hardening of the arteries in the legs causes difficulty walking with pain. The principal and most limiting symptom in PVD is intermittent claudication—pain in the legs while walking. In more severe cases, leg ulcers, and eventually amputation, may result from the peripheral vascular disease. Medications and surgery can help to restore circulation, but an important part of the medical management of individuals with claudication is exercise. Systematic review of the literature reveals that exercise is effective at increasing pain-free walking and also in prevention of more advanced disease.[22] These supervised exercise programs had success even though they usually only had three exercise sessions per week. The exercise was a program of gentle progressive walking on a treadmill for twenty to thirty minutes at a session. Even with this gentle program, a treadmill-walking test shows statistically significant and clinically relevant differences in improvement of maximal treadmill walking distance in multiple studies. The improvements are also better with a supervised exercise program than for a nonsupervised program. The average increase in walking distance was approximately 150 meters in the supervised group.[22] This is a very important improvement, as most of the subjects could only walk pain free for 200 meters before exercise and the peak mean distance was about 300 meters. This effectively means that exercise with a treadmill in a supervised setting can nearly double pain-free walking distance in people with claudication, increasing total walking distance by 50 percent. Nonsupervised exercise programs did not have nearly the same improvements. There are several possible reasons that the supervised exercise was better than the nonsupervised exercise, and key among them is that supervised exercise was generally done with a treadmill at a higher intensity than flat level ground walking done in most unsupervised programs. This is due to a dose response—a more vigorous program yields better results. Since PVD is often associated with silent cardiac disease, the cardiac mortality for individuals with claudiacation is as high as 30 percent in five years.[23–25] Fortunately, regular walking is known to decrease cardiac events,[26,27] and since the treatment of claudication includes regular walking, a significant side benefit of a walking program for claudication may be a decrease in cardiac mortality.

In view of the clear benefits of supervised exercise in claudication, a good compromise to the usual practice of advising a self-directed walking program for individuals with claudication will be to consider a supervised program to start with, and once the patient is independent, to transition to a self-directed program. Hopefully, the benefits of increased pain-free walking alone will be a motivator for patients to continue to exercise after the direct supervision ends.

Benefits of Exercise in Cerebrovascular Disease

Although most people do not think to include stroke when they think of cardiovascular disease, stroke is one of the main conditions that the American Heart Association (AHA) follows. In fact, the general consensus guidelines regarding stroke prevention is created by the AHA.[1] Among the many risk factors for stroke, the most important are primary cardiac vascular disease, peripheral vascular disease, and inactivity. The presence of coronary artery disease alone creates a relative risk of having a stroke of 1.55 to 1.73 with a 4−6 percent portion of the total risk of having a stroke.[28] Peripheral vascular disease adds 3 percent to the total risk.[1] Physical inactivity is the most important modifiable risk factor, with a prevalence of 25 percent in the general population, and is 30 percent of the total risk for stroke. Inactive people have a relative risk ration of 2.7 times active people of having a stroke.[29] In simpler terms, nearly 40 percent of the risk of having a stroke is due to inactivity, coronary artery disease, and peripheral vascular disease. Other risk factors include obesity, hypertension, diabetes, and dyslipidemia. Fortunately, these are all conditions that exercise will modify. This interaction between activity and many of the important modifiable risk factors for stroke probably accounts for the high impact on risk that is seen with inactivity.

The type of activity that can help to decrease risk of stroke is similar to that for claudication or within the recommended national guidelines for reducing cardiac risk. A daily program of thirty minutes of moderate exercise should suffice to improve risk and will help to modify blood pressure, lower lipids, and help to control diabetes and obesity. The benefits of exercise in stroke prevention have been seen in all racial and ethnic backgrounds, in men and women, in older and younger populations. The Framingham Heart Study, Honolulu Heart Program, and Oslo Study[30−32] showed protective effects of activity for men, and The Boston Nurses Health Study and the Copenhagen City Heart Study[33,34] demonstrated benefits for women. Although the dose-response data is limited, in the Northern Manhattan Stroke Study, there is clear evidence that intensive activity provided additional benefit in stroke prevention, particularly with increased duration of exercise activity.[35] Direct benefits of exercise include decreased plasma fibrinogen and platelet activity. This means that the platelets are less likely to create an unwanted clot in arteries, decreasing the risk of a stroke. Exercise also improves high density lipoproteins (HDL) that is a desired form of "good" cholesterol. Finally, exercise increases tissue plasminogen activator activity, which helps to prevent blood vessel injury.[36–38] The contribution to risk reduction is likely mediated in part by the benefit of activity in ameliorating other risk factors, such as blood pressure, diabetes, and obesity.

In established cerebrovascular disease, exercise is an important part of a secondary prevention program. The benefits include improved lipid profile, decreased blood pressure, and improved diabetes control. There is a standing recommendation for increased activity in the CDC and the AHA guidelines, and even light to moderate activity can help to reduce risk of both primary and recurrent events.[1,39,40]

Benefits of Exercise in Cardiac Disease

Primary Prevention

Just as in peripheral vascular disease and cerebrovascular disease, exercise, even to only a moderate level, can cause a significant reduction in the incidence of cardiac disease. The American College of Sports Medicine (ACSM) guidelines call for a program of exertion that is twenty to sixty minutes a day for three to five days a week.[41] Other studies have looked at levels of exercise that would be even less time demanding, in order to allow for better adherence to an exercise regimen in a busy lifestyle. In an attempt to decrease the total time commitment for exercise benefits, a study was done in 2004 to see if lower levels of exercise also had a benefit. Unfortunately, the results of this study demonstrated that the accumulation of sixty minutes of walking a week with three days of a single twenty-minute or two ten-minute bouts failed to ameliorate cardiovascular risk or to improve adiposity, blood pressure, lipids, or conditioning.[42] This implies that the level of exercise needed for cardiovascular risk modification does need a higher commitment to exercise than just a casual occasional walk, and that the ACSM guidelines should be followed. All adults should seek to incorporate the ACSM level of exercise in to their daily lives because the long-term benefits in cardiovascular prevention make the investment in exercise worthwhile.

Secondary Prevention

The role of cardiac rehabilitation in the management of individuals after a cardiac event have been well established. In 2002, the AHA released a scientific statement in support of cardiac rehabilitation as effective secondary prevention in individuals aged >75 years.[43] Unfortunately, due to a number of issues, the delivery of these services to the elderly population has lagged behind the delivery of cardiac rehabilitation to younger populations. Even among younger survivors of coronary artery disease (CAD), there is only about 50 percent attendance at cardiac rehabilitation, and maintenance of exercise over the longer term is even more limited. This is an important issue to address, since as the population of the United States has become more sedentary, there has been an increase in the number of patients who could benefit from exercise. Cardiac rehabilitation is appropriate for multiple diagnoses, including angina (severe chest pain that radiates into the jaw, neck, and arm), post coronary artery bypass surgery (CABG), arrhythmias (irregular heart beat), and for congestive heart failure (CHF—a collection of fluid in the body as the heart is unable to pump sufficiently). For in-depth coverage of cardiac rehabilitation programs with cardiovascular heart disease, the AHA statement of 2002 provides a good overview. For older individuals, who may have some specific needs, there are several review articles that provide a good overview.[44,45] Essentially, older individuals need to have a program with gentler exercise and bear in mind the limitations that may be posed by arthritis or by neurological disease. The issues of access and cost also are important, but the greatest limitation in the older population is lack of referral and lack of belief by the patients themselves that they can actually exercise.

Over the past thirty-five years, the clear effectiveness of rehabilitation for patients with CAD has been established. A comprehensive program of cardiac rehabilitation now includes risk factor modification and patient education in addition to aerobic exercise and muscular strengthening. Recent literature has demonstrated a variety of positive outcomes from these programs, including improved exercise tolerance, skeletal muscle strength, psychological status, and quality of life. Combined exercise and risk intervention programs can effectively reduce health care costs and hospitalization.[43] Despite this volume of evidence, cardiac rehabilitation is often underutilized, especially for the elderly, and especially so for women.[44,45] A key element in these programs is smoking cessation, a topic that is not discussed here, but is as important as exercise in the prevention of all forms of cardiovascular disease.

Cardiac rehabilitation for CAD patients reduces mortality by as much as 25 percent. The improvements in mortality rates are even better for CAD patients with multifactorial interventions than in patients exposed to exercise only.[43] While reduction in morbidity with cardiac rehabilitation is not clearly proven, it is important to stress that exercise training does not result in an increase in complications or illnesses.[43] Additionally, exercise has been shown to be safe with low nonfatal cardiovascular event rates. Individuals in a supervised program have a very low chance of any cardiac events, and the improvements in well-being are clearly more important than any small risk.

Emerging evidence indicates that aside from the direct benefits of exercise interventions of a cardiac rehabilitation program, intensive lifestyle modification may slow or reverse CAD in addition to the already proven benefits of exercise in lowering CAD. A patient who is committed to exercise intervention is likely to also participate in the lifestyle modifications and increase the effectiveness of other treatments for his or her cardiac disease. However, the magnitude of all the separate effects has been hard to isolate from the confounding contributions of dietary changes and lipid-lowering agents.

Energy expenditures as low as ~1,800 kcal/week, or nearly four hours of moderate physical exercise, well below the threshold of most supervised exercise intervention programs, can be effective in reducing cardiac mortality.[43]

The general principles of cardiac rehabilitation are covered in both textbooks and review articles. Special considerations should be given for special populations, including the elderly—where there should be a focus on education, medication management, and compliance—and the disabled.[43] In general, all older populations should avoid excessive impact exercises such as jogging and high impact aerobics as they are more likely to cause orthopedic issues.[43]

GENERAL GUIDELINES FOR EXERCISE

In primary prevention in healthy individuals, a brief review of some basic physiology is essential to help understand the design of a safe exercise program. These guidelines also apply to individuals with cardiac disease. A list of some of these terms and their use in cardiovascular exercise is presented here.

Aerobic Training

Aerobic training describes the exercises that increase cardiopulmonary capacity. The basic principles of aerobic training are divided into four areas: intensity, duration, frequency, and specificity (the type of aerobic exercise).[46,47] Examples of aerobic exercise include walking, running, stair climbing, cycling, cross country skiing, long distance swimming, and other sustained activity that causes the heart rate to be increased for a long period of time.

Intensity of training is defined by the intensity of the exercise performed. A program of exercises may be aimed at a target heart rate or at a level of exercise intensity such as a speed and incline setting for a treadmill exercise. A target heart rate is often used for simplicity in guiding an exercise prescription for individuals. In healthy individuals, it can be set at 80–85 percent of the maximum heart rate determined on a baseline exercise tolerance test (ETT) or an age predicted maximum. Exercises that evoke 60 percent or more of the maximal heart rate have at least some training effect.

Duration of training in the usual exercise program is twenty to thirty minutes, excluding a five- to ten-minute warming up period before exercise and a similar cooling down period after exercising.

Frequency of training is usually expressed in sessions per week. At a minimum, training programs should be done three to five times per week.

Specificity of training refers to the performance of activities in training that are the same as those desired. This is also referred to as the law of specificity of conditioning, and is commonly referred to in cardiac conditioning programs.[48] In other words, you get what you train for—that is, if you use swimming as a form of aerobic training, the benefits do not fully carry over to running, and vice versa.

The effects of aerobic training are seen in a number of physiologic parameters. These are discussed below.[47]

> *Aerobic Capacity*—The aerobic capacity (VO2Max) measures the peak capacity of the individual. VO2Max will increase with training. For example, when Lance Armstrong, one of the greatest aerobic athletes of all time, was 34, his aerobic capacity was 84 ml/kg/min, which is more than double that of an average man of the same age.
>
> *Cardiac Output* (CO)—The maximum CO increases with aerobic training. The direct relationship between VO2 and CO does not change during training.
>
> *Heart Rate* (HR)—The HR after aerobic training is lower at rest and at any given workload. The maximum HR can be slightly raised with conditioning, but will not be the primary determinant of maximum exercise.
>
> *Stroke Volume* (SV)—The SV is increased at rest and at all levels of exercise after aerobic training. Increased SV allows for maintenance of CO at a given workload with the decrease in HR described above. For example, at his prime, Lance Armstrong's stroke volume was three times greater than the average individual.
>
> *Myocardial Oxygen Capacity* (MVO2)—The MVO2 is defined as the oxygen consumption of the heart itself. Decreasing MVO2 is where cardiac protection is achieved with exercise. With conditioning, there is a lower MVO2 at a given level of work, protecting individuals from a cardiac event.
>
> *Peripheral Resistance* (PR)—The PR is the resistance presented to blood flow in by the arteries in the body. When the blood vessels are more pliable from exercise, they can relax more and lower the PR. Lowering of PR with exercise thus lowers blood pressure and makes the stress of the heart less with any level of activity and at rest.

Through changing the heart and vascular physiology described above, two benefits of exercise training are achieved, reduced cardiac risk and improved cardiac conditioning. The reduction of cardiac has been seen in many specific groups, including in the elderly,[44] women,[49] and in post bypass patients.[50] Exercise is also a cost-effective secondary prevention for cardiovascular disease as there can be significant cost savings based upon comparison with other therapies.[51]

Cardiac Rehabilitation Programs

Cardiac rehabilitation generally follows an outline that was first described by Wenger[52] in 1971. Cardiac rehabilitation is usually divided into three phases. The first phase is the acute phase, which is the hospital period immediately following a heart attack. In primary prevention there is no need for this phase as there has not been an injury. The second phase is the training phase and the third phase is devoted to the maintenance of the aerobic conditioning gains through a program of regular exercise. Risk factor modifications are taught and reemphasized throughout all phases.

Acute Phase (Phase I)

As soon as a patient is medically stable, they are out of bed and in a chair, usually by Day 1 to 2. By Day 2 to 3, short distance ambulation can be initiated and bathroom privileges are full. By Day 4 to 5, the patient is introduced to the home exercise program, stairs, and increased duration of ambulation are encouraged, and the patient completes learning the home program and is discharged. Education about risk factor modification is introduced at this time. During this phase, cardiac monitoring is usually performed under the supervision of a trained physical or occupational therapist or nurse.[53] Heart rate after heart attack is usually kept within 20 bpm of baseline. Any decrease of blood pressure should be considered worrisome and exercise halted. The major goal of the phase I program is to condition the patient to perform activities within the range of most daily activities at home post discharge.[54]

Training Phase (Phase II)

The training phase of the cardiac rehabilitation program is started after the symptom limited full level ETT in individuals with known disease. For healthy individuals, exercise can be started at a moderate level as long as there are no known health issues. The maximum heart rate maximum is determined by the exercise test, and a program designed to achieve 85 percent of the maximum heart rate is safe in healthy or low-risk individuals. For patients with life threatening arrhythmias or chest pain, a lower target heart rate should be chosen. Even a target heart rate of 65–75 percent of maximum can be safe and effective in a regular program,[55] and target rates as low as 60 percent can still yield a training benefit. For individuals at higher risk, monitoring at each increase in activity level is appropriate.

The classic duration of a cardiac training program is three sessions per week for six to eight weeks. Obviously, this is only a start to a lifelong change in habits, but should be sufficient to get an individual off to a good start. For individuals who have a difficulty to access a traditional exercise program, there are community-based programs and home programs that have been available for decades.[56,57] In all programs it is important that self-monitoring is taught. Guidelines for self-monitoring are seen in Table 2.1. Each exercise session should begin with a stretching session, followed by a warm up session, the training exercise, and end with a cool down and stretching period. It is important to remember that conditioning benefit is related to the specificity of training and that the conditioning applies to the specific muscles exercised.

Maintenance Phase (Phase III)

Although the least discussed, the maintenance phase of an exercise conditioning program is the most important part of the program. If the one stops exercising, the benefits gained from conditioning can be lost in a few weeks.

Table 2.1
Guidelines for Self Directed Exercise[*]

Patient Guidelines	Comments

Wear proper clothing	Rubber soled, leather upper shoes
	Loose fitting comfortable garments,
	   appropriate to the ambient temperature
	Follow exertional guidelines established by
	   cardiac rehabilitation team or physician
	Follow perceived exertional guidelines
	Follow heart rate guidelines

Follow exercise guidelines	5–10 minute low intensity warm up 20–30 minute exercise at target intensity 5–0 minute low intensity cool down
Stop exercising for adverse symptoms	Cardiac symptoms —chest pain —shortness of breath —lightheadedness General symptoms —joint pains —faintness with exercise

Do not exercise while ill	Wait until two days after illness has passed
	   for minor illness
	Wait until cleared by your physician for a
	   major illness or surgery

Do not exercise in environmental
   extremes
	Avoid extreme cold
	—wear warm clothing
	—use a face mask
	—exercise indoors in winter
	Avoid extreme heat and humidity
	—lower pace
	—exercise in air-conditioned environment
	—exercise early in the morning or in
	   the evening

Do not exercise after eating	Wait two hours after meals

*You should check with your physician before starting an exercise program if you have a known cardiovascular condition, or signs or symptoms of a cardiovascular condition.

The importance of continued exercise needs to be reemphasized again and again. Not doing exercise regularly is like not taking a medication—there will be no benefit if there is no continued conditioning. The ongoing exercises should be performed at the target heart rate for at least thirty minutes three times a week, if at a moderate level. If at a low level, exercises need to be performed five times a week.[47]

IMPLICATIONS FOR THE SPECIAL POPULATIONS

The Elderly

In general, elderly individuals have more comorbidities, a greater degree of deconditioning, significantly lower exercise capacity, lower quality of life, and more depression than younger patients with cardiac disease. Still, they can often show a marked increase in capacity, on par with their younger counterparts, and can have a marked improvement in quality of life with a decrease in depression indices with a high degree of safety.[43] The major issues with cardiac rehabilitation in the elderly are mostly one of access and participation, and most importantly, lack of physician referral or prescription.

Disabled Populations

Lack of referral for cardiac rehabilitation is also one of the major hurdles that stops disabled individuals from getting started in cardiovascular exercise programs. With encouragement and with involvement, these individuals can also benefit from exercise programs and achieve important improvements in cardiovascular risk factors.[43]

Exercise is essential in treatment and prevention of cardiovascular disease and since cardiovascular disease is so very common, exercise is a high-yield intervention that can prolong life, stave off disease, and prevent recurrences. Moderate exercise needs to be taken up by every individual in order to improve the quality and the length of their lives. It is the elixir of youth, alleviating or even reversing many of the conditions of aging, such as hypertension, elevated lipids, diabetes, and obesity. Best of all, exercise can be done without much cost. It is a wonderful treatment that is in the hands of the healthy individual, requires no prescription, with little to no side effects, and no need for refills.

REFERENCES

1. Goldstein LB, Adams R, Alberts MJ, Appel LJ, Brass LM, Bushnell CD, Culebras A, Degraba TJ, Gorelick PB, Guyton JR, Hart RG, Howard G, Kelly-Hayes M, Nixon JV, Sacco RL. American Heart Association/American Stroke Association Stroke Council. Atherosclerotic Peripheral Vascular Disease Interdisciplinary Working Group. Cardiovascular Nursing Council. Clinical Cardiology Council. Nutrition, Physical Activity, and Metabolism Council. Quality of Care and Outcomes Research Interdisciplinary Working Group. American Academy of Neurology. "Primary prevention of ischemic stroke: A guideline from the American Heart Association/American Stroke Association Stroke Council" (cosponsored by the Atherosclerotic Peripheral Vascular Disease Interdisciplinary Working Group; Cardiovascular Nursing Council; Clinical Cardiology Council; Nutrition, Physical Activity, and Metabolism Council; and the Quality of Care and Outcomes Research Interdisciplinary Working Group: The American Academy of Neurology affirms the value of this guideline). *Stroke* 37 (2006):1583–1633.

00000000000000000000000000

2. Balady GJ, Williams MA, Ades PA, Bittner V, Comoss P, Foody JM, Franklin B, Sanderson B, Southard D. American Heart Association Exercise, Cardiac Rehabilitation, and Prevention Committee, the Council on Clinical Cardiology. American Heart Association Council on Cardiovascular Nursing. American Heart Association Council on Epidemiology and Prevention. American Heart Association Council on Nutrition, Physical Activity, and Metabolism. American Association of Cardiovascular and Pulmonary Rehabilitation. "Core components of cardiac rehabilitation/secondary prevention programs: 2007 update" (a scientific statement from the American Heart Association Exercise, Cardiac Rehabilitation, and Prevention Committee, the Council on Clinical Cardiology; the Councils on Cardiovascular Nursing, Epidemiology and Prevention, and Nutrition, Physical Activity, and Metabolism; and the American Association of Cardiovascular and Pulmonary Rehabilitation). *Circulation* 115 (2007):2675–2682.

3. Adams HP Jr., del Zoppo G, Alberts MJ, Bhatt DL, Brass L, Furlan A, Grubb RL, Higashida RT, Jauch EC, Kidwell C, Lyden PD, Morgenstern LB, Qureshi AI, Rosenwasser RH, Scott PA, Wijdicks EF. American Heart Association. American Stroke Association Stroke Council, Clinical Cardiology Council, Cardiovascular Radiology and Intervention Council, and the Atherosclerotic Peripheral Vascular Disease and Quality of Care Outcomes in Research Interdisciplinary Working Groups. "Guidelines for the early management of adults with ischemic stroke: a guideline from the American Heart Association/American Stroke Association Stroke Council, Clinical Cardiology Council, Cardiovascular Radiology and Intervention Council, and the Atherosclerotic Peripheral Vascular Disease and Quality of Care Outcomes in Research Interdisciplinary Working Groups: the American Academy of Neurology affirms the value of this guideline as an educational tool for neurologists." *Stroke* 38 (2007):1655–1711.

4. CDC Vital and Health Statistics. "Chapter 5: Leisure Time Physical Activity." *Health Behaviors of Adults: United States, 2002–2004* 230 (2006):41–56.

5. CDC Vital and Health Statistics. "Chapter 6: Body Weight Status." *Health Behaviors of Adults: United States, 2002–2004* 230 (2006):57–65.

6. CDC Vital and Health Statistics. "Chapter 4: Cigarette Smoking." *Health Behaviors of Adults: United States, 2002–2004* Series 10, 230 (2006):22–40.

7. CDC Vital and Health Statistics. National Hospital Survey: 2004 Annual Summary with Detailed Diagnosis and Procedure Data. Diagnoses Tables 1–24: 162 (2006):8–38.

8. Morris CK, Froelicher VF. "Cardiovascular benefits of improved exercise capacity." *Sports Medicine* 16 (1993):225–236.

9. Moreau KL, Donato AJ, Seals DR, DeSouza CA, Tanaka H. "Regular exercise, hormone replacement therapy and the age-related decline in carotid arterial compliance in healthy women." *Cardiovasc Res* 57 (2003):861–868.

10. Tanaka H, Dinenno FA, Monahan KD, Clevenger CM, DeSouza CA, Seals DR. "Aging, habitual exercise, and dynamic arterial compliance." *Circulation* 102 (2000):1270–1275.

11. Neuhouser ML, Miller DL, Kristal AR, Barnett MJ, Cheskin LJ. "Diet and exercise habits of patients with diabetes, dyslipidemia, cardiovascular disease or hypertension." *Journal of the American College of Nutrition* 21 (2002):394–401.

12. Pollock ML, Gaesser GA, Butcher JD, Despres, J-P, Dishman, RK, Franklin, BA, Garber, CE. "The recommended quantity and quality of exercise for developing and maintaining cardiorespiratory and muscular fitness, and flexibility in healthy adults." *Med Sci Sports Exerc* 30 (1998):975–991.

13. Vaz de Almeida MD, Graca P, Afonso C, D'Amicis A, Lappalainen R, Damkjaer S. "Physical activity levels and body weight in a nationally representative sample in the European Union." *Public Health Nutr* 2 (1999):105–113.

14. Davison RCR, Grant S. "Is walking sufficient exercise for health?" *Sports Med* 16 (1993):369–373.

15. Morris JN, Hardman AE. "Walking to health." *Sports Med* 23 (1997):306–332.

16. Murphy M, Nevill A, Neville C, Biddle S, Hardman A. "Accumulating brisk walking for fitness, cardiovascular risk, and psychological health." *Med Sci Sports Exerc* 34 (2002):1468–1474.

17. Yaffe K, Barnes D, Nevitt M, Lui LY, Covinsky K. "A prospective study of physical activity and cognitive decline in elderly women—Women who walk." *Arch Int Med* 161 (2001):1703–1708.

18. Boreham, CA, Ferreira I, Twisk JW, Gallagher AM, Savage MJ, Murray LJ. "Cardiorespiratory fitness, physical activity and arterial stiffness. The Northern Ireland young hearts project." *Hypertension* 44 (2004):721–726.

19. Goldstein LB, Adams R, Alberts MJ, Appel LJ, Brass LM, Bushnell CD, Culebras A, DeGraba TJ, Gorelick PB, Guyton JR, Hart RG, Howard G, Kelly-Hayes M, Nixon JV, Sacco RL. American Heart Association. American Stroke Association Stroke Council. "Primary prevention of ischemic stroke: A guideline from the American Heart Association/American Stroke Association Stroke Council" (cosponsored by the Atherosclerotic Peripheral Vascular Disease Interdisciplinary Working Group; Cardiovascular Nursing Council; Clinical Cardiology Council; Nutrition, Physical Activity, and Metabolism Council; and the Quality of Care and Outcomes Research Interdisciplinary Working Group). *Circulation* 113 (2006):e873–923.

20. Morss GM, Jordan AN, Skinner JS, Dunn AL, Church TS, Earnest CP, Kampert JB, Jurca R, Blair SN. "Dose Response to Exercise in Women aged 45–75 yr (DREW): Design and rationale." *Medicine & Science in Sports & Exercise* 36 (2004):336–344.

21. Flegal KM, Carroll MD, Ogden CL, Johnson CL. "Prevalence, and trends in obesity among US adults: 2000." *JAMA* 288 (2002):1723–1727.

22. Bendermacher BL, Willigendael EM, Teijink JA, Prins MH. "Supervised exercise therapy versus non-supervised exercise therapy for intermittent claudication." *Cochrane Database of Systematic Reviews* 2 (2006):CD005263.

23. Aquino R, Johnnides C, Makaroun M, Whittle JC, Muluk VS, Kelley ME, et al. "Natural history of claudication: long-term serial follow-up study of 1244 claudicants." *Journal of Vascular Surgery* 34 (2001):962–970.

24. Dormandy J, Heeck L, Vig S. "The natural risk of claudication: risk of life and limb." *Seminars in Vascular Surgery* 12 (1999):123–137.

25. Hooi JD, Stoffers HEJH, Kester ADM, Knottnerus JA. "Peripheral arterial occlusive disease: prognostic value of signs, symptoms, and the ankle-brachial pressure index." *Medical Decision Making* 22 (2002):99–107.

26. Izquerdo-Porrera AM, Gardner AW, Powell CC, Katzel LI. "Effects of exercise rehabilitation on cardiovascular risk factors in older patients with peripheral arterial occlusive disease." *Journal of Vascular Surgery* 31 (2000):670–677.

27. Wannamathee SG, Shaper AG. "Physical activity in the prevention of cardiovascular disease: An epidemiological perspective." *Sports Medicine* 31 (2001):101–114.

28. Lumley T, Kronmal RA, Cushman M, Manolio TA, Goldstein S. "A stroke prediction score in the elderly: Validation and Web-based application." *J Clin Epidemiol* 55 (2002):129–136.

29. Gillum RF, Mussolino ME, Ingram DD. "Physical activity and stroke incidence in women and men. The NHANES I Epidemiologic Follow-up Study." *Am J Epidemiol* 143 (1996):860–869.

30. Abbott RD, Rodriguez BL, Burchfiel CM, Curb JD. "Physical activity in older middle-aged men and reduced risk of stroke: The Honolulu Heart Program." *Am J Epidemiol* 139 (1994):881–893.

31. Kiely DK, Wolf PA, Cupples LA, Beiser AS, Kannel WB. "Physical activity and stroke risk: The Framingham Study." *Am J Epidemiol* 140 (1994):608–620 [published correction appears in *Am J Epidemiol* 141 (1995):178].

32. Haheim LL, Holme I, Hjermann I, Leren P. "Risk factors of stroke incidence and mortality. A 12-year follow-up of the Oslo Study." *Stroke* 24 (1993):1484–1489.

33. Lindenstrom E, Boysen G, Nyboe J. "Lifestyle factors and risk of cerebrovascular disease in women. The Copenhagen City Heart Study." *Stroke* 24 (1993):1468–1472.

34. Manson JE, Colditz GA, Stampfer MJ, Willett WC, Krolewski AS, Rosner B, Arky RA, Speizer FE, Hennekens CH. "A prospective study of maturity-onset diabetes mellitus and risk of coronary heart disease and stroke in women." *Arch Intern Med* 151 (1991):1141–1147.

35. Sacco RL, Gan R, Boden-Albala B, Lin IF, Kargman DE, Hauser WA, Shea S, Paik MC. "Leisure-time physical activity and ischemic stroke risk: The Northern Manhattan Stroke Study." *Stroke* 29 (1998):380–387.

36. Lakka TA, Salonen JT. "Moderate to high intensity conditioning leisure time physical activity and high cardiorespiratory fitness are associated with reduced plasma fibrinogen in eastern Finnish men." *J Clin Epidemiol* 46 (1993):1119–1127.

37. Williams PT. "High-density lipoprotein cholesterol and other risk factors for coronary heart disease in female runners." *N Engl J Med* 334 (1996):1298–1303.

38. Wang HY, Bashore TR, Friedman E. "Exercise reduces age-dependent decrease in platelet protein kinase C activity and translocation." *J Gerontol A Biol Sci Med Sci* 50A (1995):M12–M16.

39. "NIH develops consensus statement on the role of physical activity for cardiovascular health." *Am Fam Physician* 54 (1996):763–764, 767.

40. Pate RR, Pratt M, Blair SN, Haskell WL, Macera CA, Bouchard C, Buchner D, Ettinger W, Heath GW, King AC, et al. "Physical activity and public health: A recommendation from the Centers for Disease Control and Prevention and the American College of Sports Medicine." *JAMA* 273 (1995):402–407.

41. Pollock ML, Gaesser GA, Butcher JD, et al. "The recommended quantity and quality of exercise for developing and maintaining cardiorespiratory and muscular fitness, and flexibility in healthy adults." *Med Sci Sports Exerc* 30 (1998):975–991.

42. Murtagh EM, Boreham CAG, Nevill A, Hare LG, Murphy MH. "The effects of 60 minutes of brisk walking per week, accumulated in two different patterns, on cardiovascular risk." *Preventive Medicine* 41 (2005):92–97.

43. Williams MA, Fleg JL, Ades PA, Chaitman BR, Miller NH, Mohiuddin SM, Ockene IS, Taylor CB, Wenger NK. American Heart Association Council on Clinical Cardiology Subcommittee on Exercise, Cardiac Rehabilitation, and Prevention. "Secondary prevention of coronary heart disease in the elderly (with emphasis on patients > or = 75 years of age): An American Heart Association scientific statement from the Council on Clinical Cardiology Subcommittee on Exercise, Cardiac Rehabilitation, and Prevention." *Circulation* 105 (2002):1735–1743.

44. Lavie CJ, Milani RV. "Benefits of cardiac rehabilitation and exercise training programs in elderly coronary patients." *Am J Geriatr Cardiol* 10 (2001):323–327.

45. Pasquali SK, Alexander KP, Peterson ED. "Cardiac rehabilitation in the elderly." *Am Heart J* 142 (2001):748–755.

46. Bartels MN. "Cardiac Rehabilitation." In *Essential Physical Medicine and Rehabilitation*, Grant Cooper, ed. (Totowa, NJ: Humana Press, 2006): 119–146.

47. Bartels MN. "Cardiac rehabilitation." In *Physical Medicine and Rehabilitation: The Complete Approach*. Grabois M, ed. (Chicago, IL: Blackwell Science, Inc., 2000): 1435–1456.

48. Blackburn GC, Harvey SA, Dafoe WA, Squires RW. "Exercise prescription development and supervision." In *Clinical Cardiac Rehabilitation: A Cardiologist's Guide*. 2nd ed. Pashkow FJ, Dafoe WA, eds. (Baltimore, MD: Williams and Wilkins, 1999): 137–160.

49. Cannistra LB, Balady GJ, O'Malley CJ, et al. "Comparison of the clinical profile and outcome of women and men in cardiac rehabilitation." *Am J of Cardiol* 69 (1992):1274–1279.

50. Perk J, Hedback B, Engvall J. "Effects of cardiac rehabilitation after coronary bypass grafting on readmissions, return to work, and physical fitness: A case control study." *Scand J Soc Med* 18 (1990):45–51.

51. Oldridge N, Furlong W, Feeny D, et al. "Economic evaluation of Cardiac rehabilitation soon after acute myocardial infarction." *Am J Cardiol* 72 (1993):154–161.

52. Wenger N, Gilbert C, Skoropa M. "Cardiac conditioning after myocardial infarction. An early intervention program." *J Cardiac Rehabil* 2 (1971):17–22.

53. Pashkow FJ, Pashkow PS, Schafer MN. *Successful Cardiac Rehabilitation: The Complete Guide for Building Cardiac Rehab Programs*. 1st ed. (Loveland, CO: The Heart Watchers Press, 1988): 211–212.

54. Sivarajan E, Lerman J, Mansfield L. "Progressive ambulation and treadmill testing of patients with acute myocardial infarction during hospitalization: A feasibility study." *Arch Phys Med Rehabil* 58 (1977):241–244.

55. Juneau M, Rogers F, Desantos V, Yee M, Evans A, Bohn A, Haskell WL, Taylor CB, DeBusk RF. "Effectiveness of self monitored, home based, moderate intensity exercise training in sedentary middle aged men and women." *Am J Cardiol* 60 (1987):66–70.

56. Pashkow F, Schafer M, Pashkow P. "HeartWatchers—low cost, community centered cardiac rehabilitation in Loveland, Colorado." *J Cardiopulm Rehabil* 6 (1986):469–473.

57. DeBusk RF, Haskell WL, Miller NH. "Medically directed at-home rehabilitation soon after clinically uncomplicated acute myocardial infarction: A new model for patient care." *Am J Cardiol* 55 (1985):251–257.

3

Pulmonary Health Benefits

Jason E. Frankel and Nicholas S. Hill

Few diseases are as debilitating and create such difficulty for patients as those affecting the pulmonary system. Many of those affected by lung disease would like to improve their capacity for various activities, yet are so limited by shortness of breath that they feel they cannot. For some, the impairment is so severe that even the simplest daily self-care tasks, like dressing or bathing, pose a challenge.

Regimented, supervised exercise has been prescribed as a treatment for lung disease for many years. Organized exercise programs can be both safe and effective in improving breathing symptoms and increasing function. Such programs, often termed "pulmonary rehabilitation programs," have been developed and studied most extensively for people with Chronic Obstructive Pulmonary Diseases (COPD), such as emphysema and chronic bronchitis.[1,2] Patients with other lung diseases such as asthma and restrictive diseases like pulmonary fibrosis can also benefit and are frequently referred to pulmonary rehabilitation programs. In this chapter, we explain what pulmonary rehabilitation programs are, how they're constructed and how members of the rehabilitation team work together, what benefits they offer to patients with lung disease, and who should enter one.

Pulmonary Rehabilitation Programs

Pulmonary rehabilitation programs usually meet in an outpatient (medical clinic) location, but inpatient and home-based programs do exist. These programs are characterized by their multidisciplinary nature; each patient meets with a special team of professionals representing different disciplines. These teams combine their experience and skill to offer greater potential benefit to patients. The specific members of such a team vary from program to program and employ only some of these team members and consult with others as the need arises, but usually include the following:

- Physician—Directs Program, screens for appropriate patients to make certain that they on optimal medical therapy and are capable of doing the necessary exercise without harming themselves, and helps with medical problems encountered by patients

  Pulmonologist—lung specialist
  Physiatrist—rehabilitation specialist

- Therapists

  Physical—Oversees strengthening and conditioning exercises
  Occupational—Deals with special needs such as devices that assist with reaching overhead or helping patients learn how to conserve energy and makes suggestions on how the home might be easier to live in
  Respiratory—Monitors the breathing status as the patients exercise, teaches breathing techniques and proper use of inhaled medications and oxygen

- Respiratory Nurse—Can do many of the above tasks if specially trained
- Nutritionist/registered dietician—Makes suggestions on diet and how to achieve optimal weight
- Social Worker/Case Manager—Can help with emotional issues, insurance challenges, and home health needs
- Psychologist—Teaches relaxation techniques, dealing with emotional issues
- Coordinator/Business Manager—Handles financial aspects of the program

In order to achieve the best results for patients, these professionals meet regularly to create a treatment plan, to assess patient progress, and to modify the plan as needed. They may also meet as a group with the patient and/or family to foster better communication.

The patient is a key member of the rehabilitation team. Patients must commit to the program, attend each session, and actively work to improve their physical ability. They incorporate recommendations from the various professionals to create a new lifestyle that allows greater levels of physical activity. Pulmonary rehabilitation programs focus principally on the treatment of patients with COPD, since the benefits have been best demonstrated in this group of patients. For this reason, insurance companies are most likely to approve coverage for COPD patients. Even so, patients who have a pulmonary diagnosis besides COPD are often covered by insurers, particularly private insurers, with the presumption that patients with many different forms of chronic pulmonary disease still stand to benefit from a program of regular exercise and education.

TYPES OF PULMONARY REHABILITATION PROGRAMS

Pulmonary rehabilitation may be given to an individual patient or to groups of patients simultaneously. Individual programs may be preferred by occasional patients who dislike working in groups, or by those who have complicated physical therapy needs, such as a patient with a neuromuscular disease like multiple sclerosis that has caused weakness and the need for specialized attention from a physical therapist. However, most pulmonary rehabilitation programs use the group approach—supervising six or sometimes even more patients simultaneously. This is more efficient from a cost perspective and most patients prefer groups because they benefit from the shared group experience and knowledge.

Pulmonary rehabilitation can be performed in an outpatient setting, inpatient setting, or at home. Patients who are too ill to be discharged may start rehabilitation as inpatients and then continue as outpatients once they are discharged. Patients are also treated as inpatients if they are receiving a special procedure, such as transtracheal oxygen, that necessitates specialized monitoring afterwards, or if they must travel an excessive distance. Home programs have been successful in some countries like the Netherlands, but not so much in the United States, where having therapists visit a patient's home is expensive. Most pulmonary rehabilitation programs in the United States use outpatient group programs that meet two or three times weekly for six to twelve weeks.

STEPS IN A COMPREHENSIVE PULMONARY REHABILITATION PROGRAM

Most patients are referred for pulmonary rehabilitation either because they are felt to require additional time and treatment to recover from the acute illness after a hospital stay for COPD, or they have received the diagnosis from an outside physician and want to optimize their condition. Many of these will have other active medical issues, such as heart disease or diabetes. The pulmonary physician who directs the program will usually conduct a screening history and physical exam to ensure that patients are safe for participation. If necessary, this doctor can recommend that a patient have additional testing, such as an exercise stress test to make sure that there is no active heart disease, or seek further advice for treating these conditions before starting exercise. The pulmonologist may also recommend changes to a patient's medical treatments for lung disease in order to improve symptoms and allow better participation.

At this point, exercise can begin. Regular exercise sessions of sufficient intensity (the amount of exertion during the workout) and duration (the length of the workout) are the most important factors in determining whether a patient achieves better symptomatic control and improved activity levels. To this end, most programs meet two to three times a week for supervised exercise and patients are also encouraged to exercise independently at home between sessions.

A "training effect," similar to what athletes achieve through regular workouts, is thought to be the reason that patients improve with rehabilitation. Exercise intensity is most often monitored using heart rate and metabolic equivalents, or "METs." One MET is the amount of oxygen used while at rest and all other activities can be described in multiples of this amount. For example, folding laundry and other light housekeeping chores require about twice the oxygen used at rest, or 2 METs. More vigorous housekeeping, such as vacuuming or mopping floors, may take as much as three times the oxygen used at rest, or 3 METs. Vigorous walking takes 4 to 5 METs, and jogging and running 6 or more METs.

Each individual has an absolute maximum amount of oxygen they can absorb at a given time and this relates to how well the lungs and heart function. The American Thoracic Society, a prominent organization of pulmonologists and affiliated professionals, states that patients who exercise for twenty to thirty minutes at least three days per week and who achieve activity requiring 60 to 75 percent of their maximum oxygen uptake can expect improvements in their endurance for activity. Because precise measurements of oxygen uptake are difficult, most programs use METs to estimate oxygen uptake and ask patients about the amount of exertion they feel during exercises. Most patients are unable to reach their target level of exercise until they have been in the program for a while, because they have to become conditioned. For this reason, the specific exercises performed and their intensity and duration need to be modified by therapists according to each individual patient's capabilities. For patients with severe breathing impairment, the target levels may have to be reduced to be more realistic.

When designing an exercise program, special attention is given to improving a patient's ability to perform specific tasks that are difficult for them. For example, patients who become fatigued or short of breath while walking, climbing stairs, or even simply rising from a seated or lying position will focus mostly on leg endurance exercises. These include exercises on a treadmill, stationary bicycle, or elliptical trainer. Other patients have more trouble with tasks that require use of the arms like bathing, dressing, or combing their hair. Because of their lung disease, these people need to use their shoulder, neck, and back muscles to help them breathe. When they attempt activities that require these same muscles, doubly taxing them, their breathing becomes more difficult. These patients still do leg exercises to improve their overall condition, but they also perform specialized upper extremity exercises with occupational therapists to improve the stamina of these muscles. Arm cycle devices and elastic exercise bands are commonly used for this purpose.

Pulmonary rehabilitation programs are not devoted exclusively to exercise.[3] Educational sessions are offered as part of most programs. Therapists, doctors, psychologists, and nurses will provide education on how to better understand their lung disease, how their inhaled medication and pills help their disease and symptoms and how to properly use them, when and how to use oxygen, how to relax and deal with "panic attacks," how to travel or have sex with lung disease, and many other topics. Patients with lung disease often have a great deal of anxiety around their symptoms and pulmonary rehabilitation is a good time for them to speak with each other and the therapists in groups about how to improve their mental and emotional state. Patients' learning from each other is an important part of doing outpatient rehabilitation in groups.

Learning how to cope better is also an important part of rehabilitation.[1] Physical and occupational therapists will provide hints on how to set the home up to make tasks easier and more efficient. Some patients will also meet individually with a social worker or psychologist to discuss emotional issues. Social workers and case managers meet with patients and their families to assist them in ordering necessary medical equipment and serve as a liaison to insurance companies. Finally, people with lung disease are often significantly overweight or underweight. A dietician may be consulted during the program to teach patients about the effect of each extreme on lung function and their symptoms. They also counsel patients on the appropriate diet for their condition.

Although most patients seeking to enter pulmonary rehabilitation programs have quit cigarette smoking in the remote past, some continue to smoke. Some programs deny enrollment and some insurers refuse coverage until smokers have quit for at least three months. Other programs enroll such patients and provide help with smoking cessation as part of the program. The physician offers counseling and/or prescriptions for medications to help with quitting; psychologists can also offer counseling and patients are provided with information about community resources to help with quitting. Either way, cigarette smoking is obviously something to be strongly discouraged in any patient with chronic lung disease and is likely to interfere with potential benefits of the program.

Most people are enrolled in pulmonary rehabilitation for between six and twelve weeks. At various points during this time, partly because insurance companies want to see the results, patients are tested to demonstrate their progress. Some tests, such as the six-minute timed walk test or maximal exertion test, are used to objectively show functional improvements. Other tests, usually questionnaires and interviews, gauge improvements in disease symptoms and individual quality of life.

THE EFFECTS OF EXERCISE ON LUNG DISEASE—WHAT GETS BETTER?

Studies of pulmonary rehabilitation programs make one fact fairly clear: the exercises used during and after the program do not usually cause improvements in actual lung function. Rather, it seems that the beneficial effects of exercise stem from the positive impact it has elsewhere in the body. The benefits include:

- Better exercise capacity
  - Ability to walk farther in six minutes
  - Leg muscle efficiency improves
  - More leg muscle capillaries (tiny blood vessels)
  - More leg muscle mitochondria (tiny power packs in muscle cells)
- Less shortness of breath with exertion
- Better quality of life
- Less time in the hospital

Many organ systems can improve function, even in the face of low oxygen delivery. For example, large muscle groups such as those in the thigh work more efficiently after conditioning in an exercise program, able to do more with the same limited amount of oxygen. Studies on biopsies from these muscles in patients who have completed rehabilitation programs show increases in the amount of blood vessels supplying them as well as more mitochondria, the "power pack" bodies within cells that provide energy. The function of the heart also improves with exercise and the increased blood flow that results can compensate in part for poorly functioning lungs. Other favorable changes take place, as well. Patients in exercise programs are more likely to learn about healthy lifestyle changes, such as smoking cessation, better eating, and weight loss techniques. All of these, especially weight loss in overweight individuals, can ease the work necessary to breathe.

Extensive research has demonstrated that the combined effects of all of these benefits make pulmonary rehabilitation particularly effective in the treatment of COPD.[2] In a very large study performed in San Diego, pulmonary rehabilitation led to improvements in exercise endurance, shortness of breath, and independence. Even when followed one year after the end of the program, most patients experienced sustained benefits. As mentioned above, patients did not show changes in the actual function of their lungs nor did they show improved survival, although the study would have had to enroll many more patients and extended for a much longer period of time, if they were going to see a survival benefit.

One way around the problem of having too few patients in individual studies is to analyze the combined results of many similar trials, something called a "meta-analysis." The Cochrane Group is a specialized service that performs these meta-analyses to answer many medical questions, not just those related to pulmonary rehabilitation. A Cochrane review asking about the benefits of pulmonary rehabilitation combined the results of twenty-three separate pulmonary rehabilitation studies and concluded that shortness of breath, quality of life, and exercise endurance as determined by the distance walked in six minutes are all significantly improved by pulmonary rehabilitation. The benefits were clearest for patients with severe COPD. The aggregated data also suggested that patients spent fewer days in the hospital after undergoing pulmonary rehabilitation, but they could still not detect a survival benefit.

Less data is available about the benefits of exercise for pulmonary diseases besides COPD, but it is clear that exercise is safe in these disease states. For instance, patients with asthma usually have no clear deficit in endurance or strength in between attacks. Rather, they are impaired more by the frequency and severity of their attacks. They often benefit from counseling with a nurse or therapist educator to learn how best to use their medications in conjunction with periods of exercise. One study does show that a swimming program safely improved endurance in asthmatics and also decreased the number of asthma attacks these patients experienced. On the other hand, patients with cystic fibrosis are often referred to respiratory therapists to help with lung secretion

For Patients with Asthma

Asthma is different from other lung diseases in several ways. First, asthma is not the result of damage to lung tissue because of cigarette smoking, infection or immune diseases. Rather, asthma symptoms result from unexpected tightening of the airways, which makes breathing more difficult. Asthma attacks can be provoked by many different things, such as allergic reactions, smoking, stress, and even certain forms of exercise.

Medication is the most common treatment and preventative for asthma symptoms. However, exercise is safe and healthy for people with asthma. Studies by I. Matsumoto and M.C. Weisgerber, among others, show that swimming produces fewer asthmatic symptoms than other forms of exercise and brings about similar improvements in endurance and muscle function. No study has conclusively shown that swimming can reduce the severity of asthma symptoms when they occur.

While people with asthma may not need a full pulmonary rehabilitation program, they can benefit from meetings with a pulmonologist, respiratory therapist or nurse, and even physical or occupational therapists. These people can help patients make the best use of their medications and learn what situations to avoid in order to minimize symptoms.

management, and small studies suggest that they are safely able to participate in exercise programs. Patients with bronchiectasis may have some symptomatic relief with exercise, but there is no evidence that comprehensive pulmonary rehabilitation programs hold special benefit for them. Patients with less common diseases like pulmonary hypertension (high blood pressure in the lungs) and pulmonary fibrosis (scarring in the lungs that stiffens them) may also benefit from pulmonary rehabilitation, although the appropriate studies have not yet been done to substantiate this. Thus, the types of lung diseases that can be helped by pulmonary rehabilitation are:

COPD
Asthma
Cystic fibrosis
Interstitial lung disease; pulmonary fibrosis
Lung cancer
Neuromuscular diseases like multiple sclerosis or post-polio syndrome
Before or after major surgery in patients with lung disease
Before and after lung transplantation or lung volume reduction surgery
Pulmonary hypertension

STARTING AN EXERCISE PROGRAM

Pulmonary rehabilitation programs clearly offer special benefit for patients with moderate or severe COPD, but these patients should start exercising only under the supervision of a physician and qualified professional therapists. A physician can help the patient understand their pulmonary disease and determine how much exercise is safe, taking into account heart function and overall strength to help determine a realistic starting point. Of course, a doctor can also prescribe medications and oxygen use to make breathing during exercise easier. Therapists then help patients take off from their starting point and progress safely but steadily to higher levels function. Specifically, they help find a rate of exercise that induces a training effect without placing dangerous demands on diseased lungs, a poorly functioning heart, or disused muscles. They often use medical equipment to monitor pulse, blood pressure, and oxygen levels to do this, something not available in a typical fitness center.

For patients with less severe disease or those who wish to increase the intensity of their exercise outside of a formal pulmonary rehabilitation program, it is still a good idea to consult a physician before starting. If a person has undiagnosed cardiac disease and quickly starts intensive exercise, there is a chance that placing excessive strain on the heart can cause a heart attack. The American College of Sports Medicine, which studies exercise, its risks and benefits, recommends that men over forty and women over fifty consult a physician before abruptly beginning a new exercise program. This is to determine the likelihood of heart disease in the individual and recommend whether cardiac testing is necessary. Nonetheless, there is no need to be fearful about starting an exercise program for most people because the potential gains of regular exercise far outweigh the slight risks involved. Checking with their doctor first is always safest, but starting slow and stopping if they detect body signals like excessive shortness of breath, chest pain, or dizziness is sensible. Obviously, if they experience the latter symptoms, they should seek prompt medical attention.

MAINTAINING AN EXERCISE PROGRAM

Patients who complete a pulmonary rehabilitation program usually experience measurable increases in their walking endurance and other functional measures as described above, but as in any conditioning program, once they stop exercising, they lose ground. Therefore, patients are instructed to continue at home what they learned in the pulmonary rehabilitation program; walking or stationary cycling several times weekly. Unfortunately, many patients, even with the best intentions, gradually lose interest in regular exercise and become deconditioned all over again. For this reason, many programs have started "maintenance programs" to allow patients to return to the rehabilitation center two or three times a week to exercise under supervision, getting the additional benefit of working with a group of patients with lung disease. Patients who return to these sessions appear to maintain their improvements quite well, although it has not been proven that they do better than they would have had they exercised at home. Insurance companies do not cover maintenance programs, so individuals must pay out of pocket. Most programs keep fees low, though, so that most patients can afford to come.

If no maintenance program is available or the patient isn't interested in continuing one, other considerations can be helpful in maintaining exercise beyond the end of an organized, intensive rehabilitation program. Exercise is easier to maintain when there are other benefits:

- Listening to music while exercising is a useful reward for some and can help one to maintain the intensity of the exercise regimen and stick with it for longer.
- Exercise classes at a fitness facility are often inexpensive and can provide a fun, social atmosphere, similar to that achieved at the rehabilitation center.

WHO SHOULD ENTER A PULMONARY REHABILITATION PROGRAM?

Almost any patient with a chronic lung disease and impaired function, either permanent or intermittent, stands to benefit from pulmonary rehabilitation (see Table 3.1). Because the evidence supporting the benefit of pulmonary rehabilitation is mainly for COPD, insurers, especially Medicare or Medicaid, may balk at covering patients with other diagnoses. Nonetheless, many private insurers are willing to consider coverage for patients with other diagnoses; it is certainly worth contacting them and attempting to convince them to provide coverage.

Some patients are better candidates for pulmonary rehabilitation than others because they stand to benefit more. The best candidate is someone with moderate to severe exercise impairment who has adequate residual lung capacity and is out of shape. This individual can benefit enormously from a regular exercise program. Patients who have mild disease or exercise regularly

Table 3.1
Who Should Enroll in Pulmonary Rehabilitation?

Chronic lung disease with exercise impairment
    Potential for improvement
    Motivation
    Able to comprehend instructions
    No contraindications (e.g., unstable, untreated heart or neurologic disease)
    Adequate finances
    No cigarette smoking[*]
Preoperative to enhance conditioning or postoperative to speed recovery in patients with chronic lung disease

---

[*]Medicare in some states requires three months of smoking cessation before approving coverage for rehabilitation.

already and are in good shape will benefit less, because they have less room for improvement. Patients with very, very severe lung disease will not benefit as much because they lack the lung capacity to do much exercise at all and it may be difficult to achieve a training effect. These patients are sometimes enrolled in the program on a trial basis to give them a chance and see if they can do more than anticipated.

Motivation and the ability to comprehend are also important attributes. Patients must be committed to the program. If they miss frequent sessions or don't try when they are exercising, they cannot achieve a training effect. If they are unable to comprehend the purpose of the program or follow instructions due to a psychiatric problem, brain injury, or dementia, they are very unlikely to be able to exercise adequately.

They must be medically stable in other ways to be good candidates. If they have poorly controlled heart disease and are at risk for a heart attack, or neurologic problems that predispose them to falling, fainting, or having seizures, or such bad joint problems that they can't exercise, they are obviously poor candidates unless these problems can be corrected. The physician who screens patients should detect these problems and not allow patients to start the program until they are adequately treated and stabilized.

Some insurers (e.g. Medicare) will not cover cigarette smokers unless they have stopped at least three months before program initiation and some programs independently bar smokers from participation. Of course, all cigarette smokers should be encouraged to quit, and those entering pulmonary rehabilitation that permit smokers should incorporate smoking cessation into the program.

A common reason for entering pulmonary rehabilitation is to prepare patients with lung disease for major surgery or to speed their recovery afterwards. Such surgeries include bypass surgery for the heart, abdominal aortic aneurysm repair, and others. Sometimes patients are preparing for or recovering from lung operations like lung transplantation or lung volume reduction surgery. With the latter surgery, which consists of removal of areas of lung with extensive emphysema from carefully selected COPD patients, participation in a preoperative pulmonary rehabilitation program is required by insurers.

How to Find a Pulmonary Rehabilitation Program

Primary care or pulmonary physicians may recommend pulmonary rehabilitation programs for their patients with chronic lung disease, but sometimes they are unaware of the benefits or locations of such programs. Patients with chronic lung diseases are encouraged to ask their physicians for information on local programs. If physicians lack such information, patients can locate programs by contacting local hospitals to see if they run programs or check with their local American Lung Association, which may have a list. Patients require a physician referral to begin, but most physicians will be happy to provide a referral if a patient with lung disease requests it.

Who Pays for Pulmonary Rehabilitation?

Most insurance companies will cover pulmonary rehabilitation for patients with lung disease. Guidelines for coverage vary from state to state and between different insurers, so patients should check with their insurance company to determine whether they qualify and what will be covered. Some companies have prohibitions, such as refusing to cover pulmonary rehabilitation for patients still smoking cigarettes. In general, insurance companies will not pay for maintenance programs.

Pulmonary rehabilitation has assumed an important role in the management of chronic lung diseases, especially COPD.[4] Consisting of multidisciplinary teams providing supervision mainly to outpatients in groups, pulmonary rehabilitation programs use exercise regimens and educational programs to improve exercise capacity, shortness of breath, and quality of life in patients with COPD and probably other lung diseases. Almost any patient with a chronic lung disease and functional impairment should look into the possibility of participating in pulmonary rehabilitation, determining what programs are in their vicinity, and whether insurance will cover their participation. They can learn to do things more efficiently with less shortness of breath and enhance their confidence in managing their own disease.

References

1. Ries AL, Kaplan RM, Limberg TM, Prewitt LM. Effects of pulmonary rehabilitation on physiologic and psychosocial outcomes in patients with chronic obstructive pulmonary disease. *Ann Intern Med.* 1995; 122:823–832.

2. Lacasse Y, Brosseau S, Milne S, Martin S, Wong E, Guyatt GH, Goldstein RS. Pulmonary rehabilitation for COPD. *Cochrane Database Syst Rev.* 2002:CD003793.

3. Hill NS. Pulmonary rehabilitation. *Proc Am Thorac Soc.* 2006; 3:66–74.

4. Nici L, Donner C, Wouters E, Zuwallack R, Ambrosino N, Bourbeau J, Carone M. American Thoracic Society/European Respiratory Society statement on pulmonary rehabilitation. *Am J Respir Crit Care Med.* 2006; 173:1390–1413.

4

STRENGTH TRAINING HEALTH BENEFITS

Daniel Dodd and Brent Alvar

Aerobic exercise has long been the prescriptive method for improving health, however there is now growing support for the use of resistance training as an isolated or cooperative method to aerobic training in achieving improvements in health outcomes. Within the human body, skeletal muscle accounts for 45 percent of total body weight and is the largest tissue within the human body.[1] For many years the preservation and development of muscle tissue has commonly been the focus of athletic populations and those looking to enhance their physique; however, the relationship between strong and active muscle tissue to sustaining good health is becoming much more evident. Strikingly, between the ages of 30 and 70, muscle mass and strength decrease by an average of 30 percent and has been shown to have both direct and indirect associations with a number of current health issues.[2]

Resistance training has consistently been proven as the most effective method available for maintaining and increasing lean body mass and improving muscular strength, power, and endurance,[3] yet it is inadequate levels of muscular composition and strength that have been associated with the inability to maintain and improve bone mass, decreased glucose tolerance, increases in fat mass, metabolic inefficiency, compromised musculotendinous integrity, and decreases in the ability to carry out activities of daily living.[4] These factors considered, it is disconcerting that only 21.9 percent of men and 17.5 percent of women in 2004 reported strength training two or more times a week, and the statistics are even less prevalent in those 65 years of age and older with only 14 percent of elderly men and 10.7 percent of elderly women meeting the two day per week standard.[5] It is becoming quite evident that the lack of involvement in resistance training and subsequent decreases in muscle mass and strength are being largely overlooked as a contributor to a society facing health epidemics, such as the metabolic diseases, obesity, and type II diabetes, as well as bone deterioration, cancers, and age-related loss of muscle mass and strength (sarcopenia). This chapter will provide the basic concepts of resistance training and identify the importance of including this modality into one's physical activity programs for improved muscle-related physiological patterns and overall health enhancement.

HISTORY OF RESISTANCE TRAINING

The nomenclature involving the art of lifting weights is varied with terminology such as "resistance training," "strength training," or "weightlifting" the commonly used phrases. Though these terms are basically the same, it should be acknowledged that "strength training" specifically refers to the act of lifting weights for improvement in muscular strength, "weightlifting" specifically refers athletes performing exercises specific to the sport of Olympic weightlifting, such as the Clean and Jerk and Snatch. "Resistance training," however is the generalized term that encompasses all methods specific to moving a resistance, such as isometrics, calisthenics, sport-specific exercises, therabands, weighted devices (medicine balls and kettlebells), free weights, or specifically designed machines (i.e., Nautilus). The American College of Sports Medicine (ACSM) and the National Strength and Conditioning Association (NSCA) prefer to use the term "resistance training" as it provides a generalized coverage of all exercises that may be used for improvement in health, body image, injury prevention, or increases in sport performance through the uses of a resistance.

Feats of resistance training have appeared throughout the history of most nations, the more popular evidential stories being the biblical Samson and the bull-lifting efforts of Milo, yet it wasn't until the early twentieth century that a Russian scientist, Sandow, one of the leading experts of the fitness revolution of that era, exposed strength training as a formidable component to formal fitness and health management. Sandow was heavily sought after by royalty, presidents, and rulers around the world for his scientific discoveries in health improvement and disease prevention. As a result of Sandow's work and that of many others, strength training became an important element to daily physical fitness around the world, particularly during wartime and throughout the first half of the twentieth century. However, the evolution of resistance training for health improvement observed a sharp decline in the United States during the late 1960s and throughout the 1970s with the advent of cardiovascular specialists such as Dr. Kenneth Cooper who advocated the superior benefits of aerobic exercise over resistance training on health outcomes. The following two decades led to a separation in these two types of exercise based on the reason for which they were utilized. Strength training was used primarily for the improvement of human performance in athletic and gym settings whereas aerobic training focused primarily on the improvement of the cardiovascular system and the subsequent health improvements that resulted from this form of training. It has only been in very recent times that resistance training to produce muscular enhancement and improve health has truly become a scientific discipline. The quest for superior strength has led to the discovery of numerous systems of strength training and thereby laying a solid experiential foundation for the far more refined methods of today to improve both human performance and health outcomes.[6] Although there have been advancements in scientific knowledge most of the time-honored strategies have remained in place; an arm curl is still an arm curl. Additional research is needed to determine further benefits, techniques, systems, and possible ill effects from both old and new strategies.

BASIC DEFINITIONS OF RESISTANCE TRAINING

Before discussing the use of resistance training as it pertains to health benefits it is important to define some of the commonly used terminology. Each of these terms plays a significant role in optimizing health outcomes.

Resistance training is the use of the body's musculature to move (or attempt to move) against an opposing force. It encompasses the use of free weight or weight machines and the manipulation of repetitions, sets, intensity, and rest through a wide range of training modalities for the purpose of muscular hypertrophy (increased muscle size), muscular endurance, muscular strength, or muscular power.

A *repetition* is one complete movement of an exercise and consists of two phases: the concentric muscle action, or the lifting of the resistance, and the eccentric muscle action, or the lowering of the resistance. A repetition can also include an isometric muscle action, where the tension developed by the muscle is equal to that of the resistance attempting to be overcome, in which case no movement occurs.

A *set* is a group of repetitions performed continuously without stopping and can consist of any number or repetitions, typically ranging from one through fifteen repetitions; however, though not often recommended, training for muscular endurance can often surpass fifteen repetitions.

Intensity in resistance training is often determined by a repetition maximum (RM), the maximum number of repetitions per set that can be performed at a given resistance while maintaining proper lifting technique. A 1RM is the heaviest resistance that can be fully completed only once and is categorized as maximum intensity (100 percent). Prescribing intensity is often set as an RM, such as 10RM, which denotes that the exercise is to be only be completed a maximum of ten times and the individual should choose a resistance that can only be completed the set number of times. Intensity can also be set as a percentage of the 1RM, such as 90 percent 1RM. This denotes that the individual is to lift 90 percent of the resistance that can only be lifted one time. For example, individuals may achieve a 1RM of 150lbs for the bench press exercise and if they are prescribed to train at 90 percent of their 1RM then each weight they train at for that day should equal 135lbs per set. The use of these two methods to prescribe intensity allows both the monitoring of an individual's progress throughout a training program and can help establish the necessary progression for that individual to improve on their current muscular development.

Overload. The most important facet to resistance training is through using the principle of progressive overload. For a training adaptation to occur, such as increase in muscular endurance, size, strength, or power, the physiological system must be trained, or stressed, at a level beyond what it is currently accustomed to. Adaptation in the physiological systems will continue to occur until the tissues are no longer overloaded. The type of exercise used, the duration of training, the intensity, and the frequency are all variables pertinent to progressively overloading the physiological systems.

The following terminology describes the various muscular adaptations that occur from manipulation of the aforementioned variables.

Muscular hypertrophy is the use of resistance training to create maximal activation and breakdown of muscle protein therefore resulting in the synthesis of new muscle protein and growth of overall muscle tissue, in other words, building muscle. Muscular hypertrophy is obtained by completing several exercises (two to five) for the same muscle group, of moderate (10–12RM) to heavy (5–7RM) resistances, and keeping rest intervals between sets short (one to two minutes).[7] It is suggested that training for long periods (> eight weeks) will provide maximal increases in muscle size.[8] Muscular hypertrophy is commonly sought after by those looking to improve their muscle definition and muscular physique, the extreme of which is bodybuilding and some athletic populations.

Muscular endurance is characterized by the ability of the working muscles to complete a number of repetitions (> one) to complete muscle failure, or the amount of time muscles can perform while maintaining a designated posture or speed of lifting. Training for muscular endurance is completed using intensities of between 20 percent and 80 percent 1RM to complete muscle failure.[7] The goal of training for muscular endurance is to achieve muscle fatigue and therefore sets and rest periods are arranged according to each individual's ability to withstand fatigue and muscle failure. Circuit training is the most commonly used approach to training for muscular endurance. Some endurance athletes, such as long distance runners and swimmers, typically resistance train to improve both the endurance capabilities of the muscles and the mechanical efficiency, that is, being able to perform more or same work with less energy expenditure.

Muscular strength is the maximal amount of force a muscle or muscle group can generate in a specified movement pattern at a specified speed of movement.[9] A 1RM is typically represented as an individual's maximal strength level for a given movement. Training for gains in muscular strength occurs by completing sets of heavy (< 5RM) to maximal (1RM) resistances with long rest periods (three to five minutes) between sets and working only a few exercises (two to three) per muscle group per workout. A further description of training for muscular strength for different populations will be discussed further in this chapter.

Muscular power is the product of the force applied by the working muscles on the resistance multiplied by the velocity of movement against the external resistance. More simply, muscular power is the amount of work that is completed divided by the time taken to achieve that work. Training for muscular power entails the development of both the force and the velocity component. This is achieved through the lifting of heavy resistances (for the force component) and light to moderate resistances at high movement speed (for the velocity component). The recommended training variables for muscular power development are three to five sets of one to five repetitions per exercise with rest periods of between three and ten minutes.[10] It is important in training for power that each repetition or set of repetitions be completed at maximal intensity of movement and in a fatigue-free state.

There are many different types of training that have differing desired outcome and physiological effects as discussed earlier, however, it is very important to have a working knowledge of these types so that you can differentiate between them. The following list uses many of the same exercises and equipment at times, the difference is in the desired goal, strategies of training, and the intensity and volume used (such as sets, reps, loads, etc.).

Resistance training for increases in muscle definition
Resistance training for sport (sport-specific training)
Cardiac rehabilitation resistance training
Power lifting
General resistance training for endurance, size, strength, or power
Olympic weight lifting
Bodybuilding
Rehabilitative resistance training
Functional resistance training in the prevention and control of the deleterious
    effects of disease, aging, and disability

Though all of these training modalities provide specific physiological outcomes pertinent to the focus of that modality, such as increased muscle size, endurance, or power, it is training for strength that has been shown to create adaptations across all three physiological outcomes. More importantly, training for strength has been shown to provide significant improvements over a multitude of health outcomes.

HEALTH BENEFITS OF STRENGTH TRAINING

Strength training is slowly becoming more prominent as an effective modality to improving health and more importantly in the management and prevention of disease. The major societal diseases being faced today include metabolic diseases such as obesity, diabetes, hypercholstrolemia (high cholesterol), hypertension (high blood pressure); joint and bone deterioration such as arthritis and osteoporosis; sarcopenia (loss of muscle mass and strength); and numerous variations of cancer. These conditions are all characterized by vastly different physiological symptoms and therefore a wide array of behavior modifications are needed, yet through resistance training, there is a likelihood of prevention and/or management of these diseases as well as lifestyle improvements such as activities of daily living.

Metabolic syndrome entails coexisting risk factors that place an individual at high risk for all cause and cardiovascular mortality and development of diabetes and is clinically defined as having three or more of the following criteria: abdominal obesity greater than 102cm (40 inches), high triglycerides (greater than 150mg/dL), low high density lipoprotein (less than 40 mg/dL), hypertensive (high blood pressure, greater than 140mmHg systolic or 85mmHg diastolic), a high fasting glucose (greater than 100mg/dL), and/or self-reported diabetes.[11] For such metabolic diseases as diabetes, hypercholesterolemia, and obesity the use of aerobic training has typically been advocated as the preferred method for reducing risk levels. However, more research is accumulating on the importance of resistance training in providing greater benefits in reducing these disease risks than aerobic exercise alone.[12,13] These diseases are complex, multifactor conditions with genetic, physiological, metabolic, social, cultural, environmental, and psychological components, and as such are equally complex in appropriate treatment.[10]

A less obtrusive symptom of underlying chronic disease is hypertension. Hypertension is high levels of blood pressure (greater than 140mmHg systolic or 85mmHg diastolic) and a risk factor linked to chronic diseases. If left untreated, it can be a contributor to increased morbidity and mortality. Currently, over 25 percent of Americans can be classified as hypertensive.[14] It has been shown that increased levels of physical activity, greater levels of fitness, and the use of resistance training are related to a reduction in the incidence of hypertension. Resistance training was considered contraindicated for those classified as hypertensive due to the increase valsalva pressure (forced expiration against a closed glottis can cause a dramatic increase in both systolic and diastolic blood pressure) seen during this type of exercise. In addition, it was thought that resistance training would actually chronically increase blood pressure due to vascular hypertrophy and increased vascular resistance due to large acute increases in blood pressure elicited by the exercise. Current research has begun to refute the longstanding belief of increased risk to those with hypertension. The ACSM recently recommended a resistance training program combined with an aerobic training program to help prevent, treat, and control hypertension.[15] A meta-analysis by Cornelissen and Fagard[16] found that moderate resistance exercise should be part of a nonpharmacological intervention strategy to prevent and combat high blood pressure and further suggested the additive effect if used in combination with aerobic training. It should be noted that individuals undergoing drug treatment to reduce the levels of hypertension should consult with a medical and strength training professional prior to starting an exercise program to identify the results of a combined exercise program and the response from the medication.

Along with hypertension, hypercholesterolemia is another symptomology of underlying disease progression, and similar to hypertension, there is considerable research to show the benefits of resistance training on reducing the risk of hypercholesterolemia. Fahlmen and colleagues[17] showed a favorable response to blood lipid profiles for the resistance training intervention as compared with an endurance training group or control. After ten weeks of either endurance training or high intensity resistance training the subjects experienced an increase in HDL cholesterol and a decrease in triglycerides. The resistance training group was also significantly lower in total cholesterol and LDL cholesterol as compared with the control group. Both the resistance training and endurance training resulted in favorable changes to plasma lipoprotein levels for elderly women in only ten weeks and this occurred without alteration to weight or diet. Uncontrolled hypertension and hypercholesterolemia can be a precursor to diabetes.

The incidence of diabetes, particularly type II diabetes is one disease that is increasing rapidly in both children and adults and is characterized as the inability of the body to produce or properly utilize insulin. Type II diabetes is a condition that can develop as a result of lifestyle choices, such as dietary intake (high levels of fat and sugar intake) and lack of physical activity. This results from insulin resistance, in which the body fails to properly use insulin to remove the increased glucose in the blood.[13,18] In 2003, the number of Americans classified as prediabetic reached 20 percent,[19] and following diagnosis, 75 percent of these individuals will develop type II diabetes within ten years unless appropriate lifestyle changes are made.[20] Muscular strength is inversely related to metabolic syndrome, independent of cardiovascular fitness levels, and through strength training, and the subsequent increases in muscle tissue become the primary recipient of blood glucose and fat to be used as energy, and thus lowering the levels of insulin release.[18] Muscle activity increases glucose uptake during higher intensity activities and facilitates an increased utilization of fat during lower intensity activities and while in a resting state.[11,21]

The impact of strength training on bone health is related specifically to the relationship between the increased tensile strength of the developed muscle and the strains imposed onto the structural components of the bone. Before this relationship can be discussed, it is important to understand the function of bone and how strength training becomes such an integral part of bone management. The main function of bone is to provide the mechanical integrity for locomotion and protection; accordingly, bone mass and architecture are adjusted to control the strains produced by mechanical load and muscle activity.[22] That is, the types of activity we do and the stress imposed on the bone has a direct impact on bone deterioration and more importantly, on the ability of new bone formation. The response to mechanical strain imposed on bone is site-specific and though the exact mechanisms by which muscle activity and weight-bearing can activate the adaptive processes of the bone are still unclear, it is assumed through animal studies that bone adaptation responds to specific fundamental rules.

Bone adapts more highly to dynamic, rather than static movements. Dynamic movements provide sufficient magnitudes or rate of strain and with short periods of exercise and long rest periods between them it provides more osteogenic (bone forming) stimuli. Dynamic activities, such as tennis and basketball provide substantial bone loading and create the necessary impact forces for bone reformation to occur, rather than single sustained exercises like walking that have relatively low rates of strain and produce customary mechanical loading that makes bone cells less responsive to routine loading signals and decreases the ability for bone formation.[22] Bone degeneration, such as osteoarthritis and osteoporosis, has become one of the leading health issues in older individuals (approximately 90 percent of hip fractures are from falls in the elderly) and postmenopausal women. It is the third most serious disease in the current population and affects approximately 25 million people, of which 80 percent are women. It is even more concerning that one-sixth of women who suffer an osteoporotic fracture have died within one year.[23] It is these concerns, among others, where resistance training can have a significant impact in slowing down, improving, and preventing if started at a young age. For the bone disease osteoarthritis, a painful form of degenerative arthritis that affects a low percentage of all young adults and includes the majority of all senior adults, heavy resistance training has been argued to be detrimental and often suggested could be a contributor to osteoarthritis.[24] It has been previously thought that the use of heavy resistances provides too much strain on the skeletal joints and exacerbates pain and discomfort associated with the diseases.

However, the use of resistance training, particularly heavy loads, produce more extensive compressive force that is the essential ingredient to the process of bone remodeling. This is particularly evident if the resistance training repetitions are completed to muscle failure, this may provide greater compressive forces and shear stresses on the joints.[7] Even completing a set to "volitional" failure (a point determined by the individual as their repetition end point and typically just short of complete muscle failure) may reduce the joint aches and pains during the recovery process.[7] With higher intensity resistance training, such as that imposed in training for strength (70–100 percent 1RM), bone remodeling and the prevention of bone degradation can be achieved to the highest level.

The ACSM currently recommends higher intensity weight-bearing endurance activities such as tennis; stair climbing; jogging, and activities that involve jumping such as volleyball and basketball, as well as strength training at a moderate to high intensity (in terms of bone-loading forces) two to five times per week for a total of thirty to sixty minutes per day.[25] This is concurrent with the latest research on strength training for bone health, specifically that the key important issue for prevention and management of this disease must be the weight bearing styles of lifting and that it is of moderate to high intensity. Of the recommended activities for improvements in bone health, strength training in a controlled environment may be the safest as compared to the weight-bearing endurance activities, particularly for older individuals.

Another growing concern among the elderly populations is the decrease in muscle mass and strength with age (sarcopenia). The term "sarcopenia" was first used over fifteen years ago by Dr. William Evans and Irwin Rosenberg in the landmark book *Biomarkers, the 10 Keys to Prolonging Vitality.*[26] Sarcopenia refers to an overall weakening of the body caused by a gradual, decades-long loss of muscle mass. Sarcopenia occurs moderately in 35 percent and severely in 10 percent of the U.S. population aged 60 years and older and contributes approximately $18 billion per year in health care costs. Individuals shown to have severe sarcopenia are two to five times more likely to have a disability than older adults that are within normal levels.[27] The reduction in muscle mass and strength as individuals age has significant repercussions with the ability to perform activities of daily living (ADL). The ability to perform tasks of daily living reaches a peak in the early thirties and declines with age thereafter, and although physical activity has been shown to modify the decrement, it appears to occur regardless of activity levels, and is contributed to a variety of factors: loss of muscle, muscle weakness, and increases in fat mass.[23] The loss of muscle mass and strength associated with increases in age is due to a loss of muscle fibers (muscle cells) and subsequent destruction of viable motor units (a nerve and the muscle fibers it innervates). As a result there is a loss of alpha motor neurons, a decline in muscle cell contractility, changes in hormonal factors such as androgen and estrogen withdrawal, as well as an increase in the production of catabolic factors. The end result becomes skeletal muscle weakness and increased risks of morbidity and mortality.[7]

Epidemiological research has shown that physical activity improves muscle strength, which improves mobility, and in turn decreases the risk of falls.[1] Theoretically, there is a cause and effect relationship between physical function and resistance training. The stronger you are, theoretically the greater your ability to perform activities of daily living.[24] Unfortunately, the lack of muscular strength maintenance and development has led to a variety of physical dysfunction. Through resistance training, there is the development of connective tissue (bones, tendons, ligaments, and noncontractile elements in muscle tissue) that has the direct translation toward improving joint stability, mobility, and injury prevention in individuals, particularly older adults.[7] The benefits of resistance training on activities of daily living include increases in strength, endurance, and muscle capacity; increased flexibility; greater energy efficiency; decreased stress on the heart and circulatory system; and improved self-image and confidence.[7] Conversely, the loss of muscular strength accelerates further sarcopenia and increases the risk of falls, mortality, and morbidity.[28]

There is considerable research to show the relationship between progressive strength training programs and increases in muscular strength, lean mass, and resulting improvements in functional task performance.[29] Heavy resistance training appears to have significant anabolic effects in older adults, specifically improving the nitrogen balance, which greatly improves nitrogen retention with all intakes of dietary protein.[30] This has been assumed as the difference between continued loss of muscle and the retention of protein stores, primarily muscles protein stores.[31]

The authors of *Biomarkers* and colleagues, Walter Frontera, MD, PhD, and Maria Fiatrone, MD, were one of the first research groups to suggest that muscle mass and strength can be regained, no matter what your age and no matter what the state of your body musculature before starting an exercise program. Dr. Frontera found that older subjects, ages 60 to 72 years, were able to gain both strength and muscular size from weight training. Before this study other investigators did not push their subjects hard enough, usually having them train at 30 to 40 percent of 1RM. Frontera's research group encouraged their subjects to train like younger people at 80 percent of 1RM. After twelve consecutive weeks, three days a week, their efforts paid off with daily average increase in extensors and flexors strength of 3.3 and 6.5 percent and a 12 percent collective increase in muscle mass. The amount of muscle mass increase was what would be expected in younger people following the same regimen. A follow-up study by Dr. Maria Fiatrone expanded on the past study by investigating the frail, institutionalized elderly, 87 to 96 years old. The findings were suggested to be even more startling, where subject's muscle strength almost tripled and muscle size grew by 10 percent. Since the book release strength training the elderly has become an essential part of their physical conditioning program and regularly recommended by physicians and warranted by other health professionals.

There is currently limited research on the benefits of resistance training for cancer patients, specifically those currently diagnosed, in remission, or in recovery. However, resistance training may fulfill an important role in the recovery process, as well as during treatment, both physiologically and psychologically.[32] It is often assumed that exercise, particularly heavy lifting may exacerbate symptoms, particularly in breast cancer patients. However, Cheema and Gaul[33] showed that in twenty-seven survivors of breast cancer, there were no incidents of lymphedema or other injuries, yet significant increases in full-body strength and endurance and improvements in quality of life occurred from eight weeks of resistance training. In addition, Ohira et al.[32] also found significant improvements in body composition and strength, with subsequent correlations to decreases in depression and improved quality of life over a six-month weight training intervention. In a study by Quist et al.[34] examining forty-eight females and twenty-two males (age 18–65 years) cancer patients currently undergoing chemotherapy, a progressive aerobic and resistance training program was provided over a six-week period. The results from this study showed significant improvements in body composition, aerobic fitness, and muscular strength without any adverse effects attributable to the training program. Galvao et al.[35] also showed vast improvements in strength, functional performance, body composition, balance, and a reduction in treatment side effects in older men (59–82 years) undergoing prostrate cancer treatment. These studies are demonstrations that resistance training may indeed be a valuable component at any given point of cancer treatment and can provide preservation or improvements in muscular mass and strength, and more importantly, possibly reduce side effects common to many cancer treatment approaches.

Health Benefits and Effects of Strength Training

Morphological Factors

Muscle hypertrophy (increase muscle size)
Increase in size and strength of ligaments
Increase in bone density and strength

Neural Factors

Strength increases initially due to neural factors
Increase in motor unit activation
Decrease in neural inhibition
Balance and stability
Biochemical factors
Increase in energy stores (glycogen, ATP, and CP stores)
Increase in testosterone, growth hormone, IGF, and catecholamines

Anthropometrics

Increase body weight, BMI
Increase in limb size, decrease in skinfolds
Increase in fat free mass
Decrease in relative body fat

Additional Effects

Improved bone health (osteoporosis), joint integrity (prevention of injuries, arthritis)
Metabolic rate (weight loss)
Aerobic capacity, cardiac function (cardiac rehabilitation)
Blood lipid profile
Blood pressure (effects on hypertension—positive or negative)
Low back pain
Disability (aging)
Improved performance (sports and activities of daily living)
Increase insulin sensitivity

THE PRESCRIPTION OF RESISTANCE TRAINING FOR STRENGTH AND HEALTH BENEFITS

The American College of Sports Medicine in the position stand "Recommended Quantity and Quality of Exercise for Developing and Maintaining Cardiorespiratory and Muscular Fitness"[31] recommends the use of progressive resistance training (PRT) for all individuals, regardless of health status, and defines PRT as training in which the resistance against which a muscle generates force is progressively increased over time.[31,36] The position stand suggests training one set of eight to ten exercises (involving all major muscle groups) of eight to twelve repetitions (to volitional fatigue) and be completed two to three times a week. The position stand notes that greater frequencies of training (additional training days) and additional sets and/or repetitions may elicit larger strength gains, but the magnitude of gain would be smaller. The follow-up position stand "Progression Models in Resistance Training for Healthy Adults"[37] denotes that there is a need for progressive resistance training and chronic alterations in training sets, repetitions, exercise selection, and exercise order and rest interval needs to occur to continue adaptations from resistance training, thus as training experience increases, so should the training volume.

These position stands have provided a sound basis for most individuals undertaking a strength program, however, every individual begins with a different state of health and different level of training status, and though it has been shown in a number of studies that higher intensity resistance training sessions may provide substantially greater benefits than lower intensity or aerobic training, it is important to note that individuals need to progress slowly to the point where the body is able to withstand higher intensity training. Small increases in intensity may provide many large benefits to a variety of people and therefore higher intensity resistance training may be only necessary after one becomes further trained. Because of the vast differences in individuals it is important to identify the optimal dose of resistance training that will provide the greatest strength improvements in various populations. There have been a multitude of research showing improvements in strength from similar doses of training; however it is difficult to assimilate a true dose-response from the many studies, thus the recent ACSM guidelines suggest that the eight to twelve repetitions range is still appropriate but muscular fitness can be developed simultaneously within the reasonable and common ranges of repetitions (i.e., three to six, six to ten, ten to twelve, etc.).[37]

To explore this problem, the use of meta-analytical research approaches conducted by Rhea et al.[38,39] and Peterson et al.[40,41] combined over 175 studies on strength training with various populations to attempt to identify a dose-response paradigm. The results of these meta-analyses were able to identify the approximate number of repetitions, sets, intensity, and frequency (days per week) that should be completed to optimize strength levels in individuals of varying backgrounds. The aforementioned studies showed that for beginners or untrained individuals (those with little or no training experience) it is recommended they begin with one set per major muscle group of eight to ten repetitions in the first few weeks of a resistance training program before progressing to a mean training volume of four sets per muscle group of eight to ten repetitions or 50 percent of their 1 RM. It was reported that three times per week would provide the greatest benefit for strength improvement for these individuals.

For individuals that are recreationally trained (those with strength training experience of one year or more), there is a shift in the training variables required to elicit greater strength adaptations. The total number of sets per muscle group increased to a mean of four set per muscle group and an increase in the mean training intensity from the previously recommended 50 percent 1 RM for untrained individuals to a much higher level, 80 percent 1 RM, with a subsequent reduction in training frequency from three to two days per week per muscle group. For individuals that are classed as advanced or elite in their strength training status such as athletic populations the exercise prescription progresses to a mean training volume of eight sets per muscle group with a mean training intensity of 85 percent of 1RM and a continued frequency of two days per week per muscle group. As it can be seen from the results of these studies, the more highly trained an individual becomes there is a subsequent need for increases in the amount of work (volume) and the intensity of work in order to maintain strength gains. As a result of the increases in volume and intensity, the frequency (days per week) of training is decreased. It is believed that this is needed to allow for greater recovery from the higher intensity training programs. An important factor from these studies is that a training program utilizing low volume and low intensities such as those recommended for beginners and similar to that proposed by the ACSM position stands[25,31,37] may be an important and effective starting point, but these programs become increasingly less effective as the training status of an individual progresses.

This information can be utilized as a framework for exercise prescription guidelines relative to frequency, intensity, and volume for strength straining. It gives important information relative to differences in populations (beginner to athletes) as well as explanations as to why it is necessary to chronically alter strength training programs. More importantly, it is the authors' hope that the information can be utilized as a general guideline for how to improve strength and concurrent to that described in the first half of this chapter, it can be argued that this translation in strength will lead to improvement in general health, regardless of the health condition. The emphasis on using resistance training to improve health status needs to focus on improving muscular strength, as it appears that training for strength gains provides much greater responses than muscular endurance or cardiovascular endurance training. It should be noted that including both aerobic and strength training programs in one's physical activity habits have greater benefits than only training each of these modalities by themselves.

APPLYING THE PRESCRIPTION OF STRENGTH TRAINING: NEEDS ANALYSIS AND TESTING

Before an individual can partake in a strength training program it is important that an evaluation takes place to adjudicate his or her current physical status, any injuries, illnesses or limitations, and more importantly, define the goals that the individual is looking to achieve from attending to the program. An initial assessment of an individual needs to incorporate a number of key components.

1. Obtain a thorough appraisal by a physician or sports medicine professional of the individual's health history and current health status is required to identify if there are any underlying pathologies that may put an individual at risk or inhibit the individual from undergoing an exercise program.
2. Identify the exercise history and training background, particularly the type of program, length of recent regular participation in training programs, level

of intensity involved in the program, and the degree of exercise technique experience the individual attains.

3. Meet with a strength and conditioning specialist or physical therapist and obtain a physical ability analysis to identify the starting point of the training variables load and repetitions, and the most suitable progression approach.

The NSCA recommends the use of two possible methods to determine initial strength levels.[10] The first approach is through the use of a 1RM measure. This method is typically reserved for athletic populations or those classified as trained or advanced, due to the nature and effort required of the test procedure to achieve a "true" repetition maximum. Because of the intensity of the test, there is also a decreased reliability and validity of the results of the test if performed with less able individuals as they are typically not able to perform the test correctly and obtain a maximal lift. However, if an individual is deemed capable of completing a 1RM then the selection of large muscle group and multijoint exercises, such as the bench press for analysis of upper body strength or the back squat exercise for lower body strength, are the more suitable options as they provide substantial musculature support to handle the maximal loads and decrease the risk of injury when performing the test. For novice and less advanced individuals, it is also recommended that large muscle group and multijoint exercises be used, however the selection of exercise should be less advanced and entail the use of body weight or machine-based exercises.

The second method is the use of a repetition maximum estimate. An individual may predict a "true" RM by performing an exercise to a desired number of repetitions, such as a 5RM. By doing so, there is a reduction in the risk of injury as the loads being imposed are not maximal and an individual's body may be more apt to handle the exercise intensity. This method can be more effective when testing less trained individuals as they may be unaccustomed to the exercise or test and therefore less fearful to that of lifting extremely heavy loads. It should also be noted that the further the RM is from a true 1RM, the less predictive and reliable the result. For example, a 10RM is less predictive to that of a 3RM. The guidelines for 1RM testing can be found in the NSCA's "Essentials of Strength Training and Conditioning."[10]

Once the initial screening process is completed and all variables are taken into account, it is important that the individuals follow a progressive strength training program based on those guidelines presented earlier and their training status. It is imperative that each individual starts and progresses slowly to reach more advanced levels of training, as unprepared progressions may lead to injury, exacerbation of illnesses, and possible return to pretraining status. For most individuals, large improvements can be made with small, progressive adjustments to a strength training program. With a carefully executed program, an individual will achieve significant benefits to both muscular strength levels and to improving one's health.

Ten Resistance Training Guidelines for Strength and Health Improvements

1. Consult a medical professional for clearance to begin an exercise program.
2. Meet with strength training specialist or physical therapist to identify current training level.

Untrained	Not training or just beginning (< two months) with none or minimal technique experience.
Trained	Currently training (two to six months) with basic technique experience.**
Advanced	Currently training (> twelve months) with high technique experience. Typically includes athletes or elite populations.

**It is advisable that the first several exercise sessions be closely supervised by trained professionals.

3. Identify strength training goals and progression.

Untrained	Maximum strength gains can be achieved beginning with one set at 50 percent of 1RM, progressing to four sets at 50 percent 1RM, three days per week.
Trained	Maximum gains achieved with four sets at 80 percent 1RM, two days per week.
Advanced	Maximum gains achieved with four sets at 80 percent 1RM, two days per week.

4. Technique should never be compromised. Perform every exercise in the correct manner identified by a strength and conditioning specialist.
5. Begin with basic exercises such as body weight or machine-based movements before progressing to more advanced exercises. Consult with a professional each time a progression is to be taken.
6. Perform exercises that are dynamic and rhythmic in nature.
7. Follow the rhythmic breathing pattern of inhalation during the eccentric phase and expiration during the concentric phase. Never perform an exercise while inducing a Valsalva maneuver (forced expiration against a closed glottis—a cause of dramatic and acute rises in both systolic and diastolic blood pressure).
8. Exercises should be completed pain free through full range of motion.
9. It is best to exercise with a partner for feedback, support, and for safety.
10. Utilize the principle of *overload*. Adaptations will not occur unless progressive overload is applied through manipulation of sets, reps, load, frequency, and exercise selection.

REFERENCES

1. Buchner, D. 1997. Preserving mobility in older adults. *Successful Aging* 167(4): 258–264.

2. Nieman, David. 2006. *Exercise Testing and Prescription.* 6th ed. CA: McGraw-Hill.

3. Hass, C.J., Feigenbaum, M.S., and Franklin, B. 2001. Prescription of resistance training for healthy populations. *Sports Medicine* 31(14): 953–964.

4. American College of Sports Medicine. 2006. *ACSM's Guidelines for Exercise Testing and Prescription.* 7th ed. Philadelphia, PA: Lippincott Williams & Wilkins.

5. Centers for Disease Control and Prevention (CDC). 2006. Trends in strength training—United States, 1984–2004. *Morbidity and Mortality Weekly Report* 55(28): 769–773.

6. Siff, Mel, and Verkhoshansky, Yuri. 1999. *Supertraining.* 4th ed. Denver, CO: Supertraining International.

7. Zatsiorsky, Vladimir, and Kraemer, William J. 2006. *Science and Practice of Strength Training.* 2nd ed. Champaign, IL: Human Kinetics.

8. Fleck, Steven J., and Kraemer, William J. 2004. *Designing Resistance Training Programs.* 3rd ed. Champaign, IL: Human Kinetics.

9. Knuttgen, H.G., and Kraemer, W.J. 1987. Terminology and measurement in exercise performance. *Journal of Applied Sport Science Research* 1: 1–10.

10. Baechle, Thomas, and Earle, Roger. 2003. *Essentials of Strength Training and Conditioning.* Champaign, IL: Human Kinetics.

11. Jurca, R., Lamonte, M.J., Barlow, C.E., Kampert, J.B., Church, T.S., and Blair, S.N. 2005. Association of muscular strength with incidence of metabolic syndrome men. *Medicine and Science in Sports and Exercise* 37: 1849–1855.

12. Fahlman, M.M., Boardley, D., Lambert, C.P., and Flynn, M.G. 2002. Effects of endurance training and resistance training on plasma lipoprotein profiles in elderly women. *Journal of Gerontology* 57A(2): B54–B60.

13. Ibañez, J., Izquierdo, M., Argüelles, I., Forga, L., Larrión, J.L., García-Unciti, M., Idoate, F., and Gorostiaga, E.M. 2005. Twice-weekly progressive resistance training decreases abdominal fat and improves insulin sensitivity in older men with type 2 diabetes. *Diabetes Care* 28(3): 662–667.

14. Simão, R., Fleck, S.J., Polito, M., Montiero, W., and Farinatti, P. 2005. Effects of resistance training intensity volume and session format on the postexercise hypotensive response. *Journal of Strength and Conditioning Research* 19(4): 853–858.

15. American College of Sports Medicine Position Stand. 2004. Physical activity and bone health. *Med Sci Sports Exerc* 36: 1985–1996.

16. Cornelissen, V.A., and Fagard, R.H. 2005. Effect of resistance training on resting blood pressure: A meta-analysis of randomized controlled trials. *Journal of Hypertension* 23: 251–259.

17. Fahlman, M.M., Boardley, D., Lambert, C.P., Flynn, M.G. 2002. Effects of endurance training and resistance training on plasma lipoprotein profiles in elderly women. *Journal of Generontology* 57(2): B54–B60.

18. Ishii, T., Yamakita, T., Sato, T., Tanaka, S., and Fujii, S. 1998. Resistance training improves insulin sensitivity in NIDDM subjects without altering maximal oxygen uptake. *Diabetes Care* 21(8): 1353–1355; Albright, A., Franz, M., Hornsby, G., Kriska, A., Marrero, D., Ullrich, I., Verity, L. American College of Sports Medicine Position Stand. 2000. Exercise and type 2 diabetes. *Med Sci Sports Exerc* 32: 1345–1360.

19. Knowler, W.C., Barrett-Conner, E., Fowler, S.E., Hamman, R.F., Lachin, J.M., Walker, E.A., and Nathan, D.M. 2002. Reduction in the incidence of type 2 diabetes with lifestyle intervention or metformin. *New England Journal of Medicine* 346: 393–403.

20. American Diabetes Association. 2002. Standards of medical care for patients with diabetes mellitus: Position Statement. *Diabetes Care* 25(1): S33–S49.

21. Boer, N.F., FitzGerald, S.J., Barlow, C.E., Blair, S.N., Robertson, R.J., Kriska, A.M. 1999. Strength, weight training status, and fasting glucose in healthy adult population. *Medicine and Science in Sports and Exercise* 31(5), Supplement S85.

22. Suominen, H. 2006. Muscle training for bone strength: Review article. *Aging Clinical and Experimental Research* 18(2): 85–93.

23. Hunter, G.R., McCarthy, J.P., and Bamman, M.M. 2004. Effects of resistance training on older adults. *Sports Med* 34(5): 329–348.

24. Alvar, B.A. 2007. *Health Related Benefits of Resistance Training. Gana Salud Conference.* Madrid, Spain. In Press.

25. American College of Sports Medicine Position Stand. 1998. Exercise and physical activity for older adults. *Med Sci Sports Exerc* 30: 992–1008.

26. Evans, William, and Rosenberg, I. 1992. *Biomarkers; the 10 Keys to Prolonging Vitality.* New York: Fireside, Simon and Schuster.

27. Janssen, I., Heymsfield, S.B., and Ross, R. 2002. Low relative skeletal muscle mass (sarcopenia) in older persons is associated with functional impairment and physical disability. *Journal of the American Geriatrics Society* 50: 889–898.

28. Metter, E.J., Talbot, L.A., Schrager, M., and Conwit, R. 2002. Skeletal muscle strength as a predictor of all-cause mortality in healthy men. *J Gerontol A Biol Sci Med Sci.* 57(10): B359–B365.

29. Landers, K.A., Hunter, G.R., Wetzstein, C.J., Bamman, M.M., and Weinsier, R.L. 2001. The interrelationship among muscle mass, strength, and the ability to perform physical tasks of daily living in younger and older women. *J Gerontol A Biol Sci Med Sci.* 56(10): B443–B448.

30. Evans, W. 1997. Functional and metabolic consequences of sarcopenia. *Journal of Nutrition* 127: 998S–1003S.

31. American College of Sports Medicine Position Stand. 1998. The recommended quantity and quality of exercise for developing and maintaining cardiorespiratory and muscular fitness, and flexibility in healthy adults. *Medicine and Science in Sports and Exercise* 30(6): 975–991.

32. Ohira, T., Schmitz, K.H., Ahmed, R.L., and Yee, D. 2006. Effects of weight training on quality of life in recent breast cancer survivors: The Weight Training for Breast Cancer Survivors (WTBS) study. *Cancer* 106(9): 2076–2083.

33. Cheema, B.S.B., and Gaul, C.A. 2006. Full-body exercise training improves fitness and quality of life in survivors of breast cancer. *Journal of Strength and Conditioning Research* 20(1): 14–21.

34. Quist, M., Rorth, M., Zacho, M., Anderson, C., Moeller, T. Midtgaard, J., and Adamsen, L. 2006. High-intensity resistance and cardiovascular training improve physical capacity in cancer patients undergoing chemotherapy. *Scand. J. Med. Sci. Sports* 16(5): 349–357.

35. Galvao, D.A., Nosaka, K., Taafe, D.R., Spry, N., Kristjanson, L.J., McGuigan, M.R., Suzuki, K., Yamaya, K., and Newton, R.U. 2006. Resistance training and reduction of treatment side effects in prostrate cancer patients. *Med Sci Sports Exerc* 38(12): 2045–2052.

36. Albright, A., Franz, M., Hornsby, G., Kriska, A., Marrero, D., Ullrich, I., and Verity, L. American College of Sports Medicine Position Stand. 2000. Exercise and type 2 diabetes. *Med Sci Sports Exerc* 32: 1345–1360.

37. American College of Sports Medicine Position Stand. 2002. Progression models in resistance training for healthy adults. *Medicine and Science in Sports and Exercise* 34(2): 364–380.

38. Rhea, M., Alvar, B., and Burkett, L. 2002. Single versus multiple sets for strength: A meta analysis to address the controversy. *Research Quarterly for Exercise and Sport* 73: 485–488.

39. Rhea, M., Alvar, B., Burkett, L., and Ball, S. 2003. A meta-analysis to determine the dose response for strength development. *Medicine and Science in Sports and Exercise* 35: 456–464.

40. Peterson, M., Rhea, M., and Alvar, B. 2004. Maximizing strength development in athletes: Meta analysis to determine the dose-response relationship. *Journal of Strength and Conditioning Research* 18(2): 377–382.

41. Peterson, M., Rhea, M., and Alvar, B. 2005. Applications of the dose-response for muscular strength development: A review of meta-analytic efficacy and reliability for designing training prescription. *Journal of Strength and Conditioning Research* 19(4): 950–958.

5

FLEXIBILITY HEALTH BENEFITS

Jason E. Frankel

For centuries, many cultures have incorporated flexibility work into exercise regimens. Since ancient times, yoga practice in India has combined stretching with meditation and controlled breathing to improve physical and mental health. East Asian cultures have integrated stretching into Tai Chi and Qi Gong exercise, which guides individuals through a set of fluid motions to improve balance, strength, and confidence. Western countries usually include flexibility exercises as part of strengthening and aerobic workout routines.

Flexibility is *the extent to which certain tissues in the body can change their length safely and comfortably.* It can be measured around any joint using an instrument called a goniometer. Flexibility decreases naturally with inactivity and with advancing age. Specifically, inactivity fosters "cross-linking," or binding, of the proteins that compose muscle, tendons, and ligaments. In the short term, these cross-links are reversible. With time, they become more permanent and the natural extensibility of these tissues is reduced. With age, the production of collagen, elastin, and other proteins composing muscle and connective tissues decreases. Moveable tissues therefore do not spring back to their normal shape easily and may become more easily cross-linked. Stretching is an important tool by which these changes can be forestalled and even reversed.

This type of exercise is thought to change the extensibility of joints in a variety of mechanisms. First, stretching reverses some of the cross-links between muscle proteins, allowing greater movement. Intense, prolonged stretching may stimulate muscles to create more fibers and become larger, but it is not certain that brief, routine stretching can do this. Muscles also have built into them "spindle fibers," which provide feedback about the amount of strain on muscles. This feedback is used by the nervous system to create opposing forces in the form of a "reflex." Flexibility exercises reduce the reflex response and may thereby make it easier to move a muscle.

While stretching exercises are not as closely studied as other modes (such as cardiovascular or strength training), recent research identifies several ways that this type of exercise can add to overall health. In summary stretching may:

- help prevent injuries such as falls and muscle sprains
- lessen arthritis aches and pains
- improve mood
- allow people with preexisting diseases, such as stroke or other disabilities, to become more independent

Stretching exercise involves moving a joint through its range of motion (the natural limits of movement encompassed by that joint) in order to create a sense of "stretching" in the muscles and other tissues that support it. The American College of Sports Medicine (ACSM) defines two main types of flexibility exercise:

- *Static* (still) stretching involves moving a joint or joints to an extreme that creates the greatest elongation of a muscle or group of muscles that move the joint. The pose is usually held for fifteen to twenty seconds and may be repeated several times. A good example of this is the "hurdler" stretch, where one leg is placed straight in front of the body and the other bent at the knee alongside it. One then leans over towards the foot of the extended leg to create a gentle sense of stretching in the hamstring muscles at the back of the thigh.
- *Dynamic* stretching is accomplished by moving a joint continuously and repeatedly through its range of motion. Arm and neck circles are a common sort of slow dynamic stretching in Western culture. More elaborate forms of dynamic stretching exist in Eastern cultures, such as Tai Chi. "Ballistic" stretching is another form of dynamic stretching, in which a joint is repeatedly and forcibly propelled through its extreme of range. In some studies, these "bouncing" stretches lead to injury and for this reason are not routinely recommended. Another dynamic stretching form known as "proprioceptive neuromuscular facilitation" is described later in this chapter.

The ACSM states that anyone may benefit from flexibility exercises, no matter how old or young, and no matter how aggressively one exercises. They stress, however, that stretching alone may not be sufficient exercise to improve health. Recommendations for how to incorporate stretching into a workout are as follows:

POSSIBLE USES FOR AND BENEFITS OF FLEXIBILITY EXERCISE

Prevention of Injury to Muscles

The image of an athlete or team stretching on the field prior to a game or track meet is certainly familiar to most. Who knows for how long runners and others have been encouraged to maintain flexibility or in how many different cultures? In modern day society, athletes are certainly expected to "stretch out," both before and after any activity, and usually use both static and dynamic techniques. The exercises are thought to prevent injury, especially muscle strains and tears. Until recently, little systematic research was done to explore this notion.

Surprisingly, one recent study shows that while flexibility exercises may in fact prevent injury, they might also have associated risks. Fox example, highly skilled ballet dancers must have unparalleled flexibility for certain poses. C. Askling and colleagues surveyed ninety-nine student dancers at a prominent northern European academy over time and found that over 50 percent of students had strained a hamstring muscle within one year prior to the survey. In fact, 88 percent of those injured felt they had injured the muscle *during* a stretching activity. All reported a significant amount of time required to heal the sprain, sometimes months or even years.

This example may make one cautious about stretching, but it is wise to consider that ballet is a sport where flexibility itself matters a great deal. What of activities where flexibility is not as important to the sport? B. Dadebo and coauthors studied professional English soccer players and found that stretching may also be implicated in hamstring injuries with these athletes. Only 11 percent of those surveyed reported injury, however, and it seemed more likely to happen in those who were not supervised while stretching. As a matter of fact, when a physician, physical therapist, or professional athletic trainer was available to create a "standardized stretching program" and instruct players in how to safely perform the exercises, injuries were significantly less likely to occur.

It would seem there is no one ideal way to perform stretching exercises. The real issue is how to develop a safe, yet effective program. Many small studies exist to address this question. The most systematic found in this review was by authors Roberts and Wilson. They assigned athletes to one of three groups, which differed only by the length of time for which a series of common stretches were held. Their findings suggest that a hold time of fifteen seconds is adequate to create a measurable change in range of motion. Longer hold times did not create greater changes in range. While safety was not specifically studied, the authors reported no injuries associated with the duration of stretch in any group.

The current studies do not convincingly show that stretching alone prevents injuries in young, athletic persons. One large study by Pope and colleagues studied Australian army recruits, who either stretched for five minutes during training sessions or did not stretch at all. They report that stretching could only account for a 5 percent reduction in the likelihood of injury. When taking into account how many recruits train each year, they project that stretching alone is not a time-efficient means of preventing injuries in this population. Whether this applies to other training situations is less clear. Still, the results are compelling because the study included over 1,500 subjects.

Prevention of Falls and Improved Balance

Numerous studies examine the effects of stretching exercise on balance and the likelihood of falls in the elderly. While most of these studies followed small numbers of patients, their innovative measurement of benefits allowed them to demonstrate some significant effects.

D. Benedetto and colleagues examined the effects of yoga, a static stretching exercise program, on the range of motion about various joints crucial to walking. They also studied the changes that occurred in the characteristics of walking itself. The study showed improvements in many of these parameters. On the whole, the elders studied were younger than those in studies of other exercise programs and had very few preexisting disabilities. Only twenty-three participants were studied and no comparison group of persons using other stretching techniques or not stretching at all was included, but many changes were significant from start to finish. Most importantly, the subjects enjoyed the program and felt more confident on their feet after participating in a flexibility program.

Tai Chi is an Asian exercise discipline that uses complex, dynamic stretching to improve range of motion. Several research groups have done studies to show the benefits of Tai Chi. Drs. William Tsang and Christina Hui-Chan studied a group of twenty to twenty-five experienced Tai Chi participants, comparing each individual to someone of the same gender and similar age, weight, height, and daily level of activity, who did not practice Tai Chi. Compared with the non-Tai Chi group, those who engaged regularly in the discipline performed better in strength, balance, and position sense measurements.

A large and well-designed study by F. Li and others studied relatively inactive patients aged 72 to 90 and compared people who practice Tai Chi to those engaged in other, traditional Western stretching programs. Participants in both exercise types were organized into groups that met regularly and stretched together, in order to ensure that subjects engaged in similar amounts of flexibility exercise. The study ran for six months and individuals were regularly assessed for improvements. There was also a follow-up exam performed six months after the end of the exercise program. Tai Chi participants showed greater improvements in balance measures overall during the exercise program and maintained more of the benefits six months after completing the formal program. An important finding in this study was that Tai Chi participants reported less than half as many falls as conventional stretchers six months after the study ended.

Improving Self-Esteem and Mood

Many cultures combine stretching with meditation to bring about improvements in mood and other aspects of living. While Western society has not undertaken extensive studies to demonstrate such effects with stretching exercise alone, some small but promising studies suggest that they may exist.

R. Motl and other authors studied older adults with depressive symptoms, comparing a program of stretching and mild strength training with an aerobic walking program to determine the relative effects of each on mood. The authors reported that the two programs were comparable in their effects on depression and body image. Two weaknesses of the study are its limitation to elderly subjects and that it did not isolate flexibility exercises from other forms of exercise in order to show the effects of stretching alone. Still, older adults desiring to improve their moods who are not able to move easily enough to walk long distances should be encouraged that even a less intensive and largely immobile exercise program may prove beneficial to them.

Yoga has been studied periodically for its potential to improve mood and physical disability in people who have been treated for cancer. Studies are too small to show consistent benefits, but a study by S.N. Culos-Reed and colleagues suggests it may create significant improvements in quality of life measures, emotional function, and post-chemotherapy and radiation therapy diarrhea. The authors assert that "alternative" exercise programs, like yoga, have major advantages in encouraging cancer survivors to become more physically active. Yoga "asanas," or poses, can be modified and slowly advanced to full form as a student gradually improves. This is useful for patients who have just finished chemotherapy, radiation, or have recently had surgery, and are either incapable or wary of participation in more aggressive exercise because of the physical demands.

Improving Disability

Research studies are hardly necessary to prove the benefits of stretching in individuals who have had strokes, physical trauma, amputation, and countless other disabling illnesses. Where there is muscle weakness or a change in the architecture of joints, cross-linking occurs and permanent alterations in range of motion, termed "contractures," may result. Contractures can worsen disability by preventing movement such as reaching over one's head to put on a sweater or bending a hip and knee enough to take a step while walking. Flexibility training, both with and without the help of a professional therapist, has long been the standard treatment for contractures. It can both enhance function and reduce the amount of energy required to perform a task, allowing the disabled person greater mobility and independence. In cases where paralysis or mental awareness prohibits independent function, increasing flexibility may ease demands on caregivers who routinely perform these tasks for others.

A special problem affecting those with injury to the brain or spinal cord is uncontrollable muscle spasms called *spasticity*. In addition to being uncomfortable, spasms may worsen contractures or prevent the voluntary use of muscles that otherwise have enough strength for useful activity. Frequent stretching is the first-line therapy for spasticity. In cases where stretching alone does not reduce the spasms to acceptable levels, it may be combined with medication or special surgical procedures.

There are also special techniques used by therapists to augment stretching exercises, such as the application of ice, splints, and mild electrical currents to the affected region. For patients with especially stubborn spasms, a highly specialized stretching technique called *proprioceptive neuromuscular facilitation*

(PNF) is used. In PNF a skilled therapist moves the joint passively until the point of spasm is reached, then uses voluntary activation of other muscle groups to reduce the contraction of the spastic muscle. The joint is then more easily and aggressively stretched.

While initially developed for those with muscle spasms, PNF can also be used in athletes and others who require greater range of motion. It more rapidly improves flexibility, but is a cumbersome method that requires a skilled trainer or therapist to apply. Most athletes will find other static and dynamic stretching techniques more convenient and nearly as effective over time.

Improving Pain

While forcible movement around a painful joint may be the last thing one would desire, aggressive stretching can be an important part of the treatment for conditions such as chronic low back and joint pain. Whether the cause is a severe muscle strain, arthritis, a pinched nerve, general weakness from decreased activity levels, or musculoskeletal injury due to years of demanding physical labor, flexibility is almost always incorporated into treatment. Stretching may help joints to move and work together more efficiently, decreasing pain. No one is exactly sure of the mechanism by which stretching helps alleviate discomfort, but just as with athletes, supervised dynamic and static flexibility exercises have analgesic effects.

Stuart McGill, PhD, a well-known authority on disorders of the back and author of a commonly referenced book on the subject, has reservations about stretching alone for low back pain. He alludes to research showing that patients with very flexible spines but significant weakness in the back muscles reported more pain and problems with their backs. He therefore believes that stretching should never be prescribed for low back pain without first strengthening damaged muscles to ensure the stability of the spine. Some exercises, especially those that bend the spine forward, may also transiently worsen symptoms resulting from bulging discs and compressed nerves. Patients with chronic low back pain are thus well-advised to seek help from a health professional before engaging in aggressive stretching activities. A physician, trainer, or professional therapist can help identify which, if indeed any, specific muscle groups require greater mobility and recommend appropriate measures.

The complaint that aggressive stretching only makes the underlying pain worse is all too familiar to health care workers. Patients for whom stretching at any level is too uncomfortable should explore options for pain management with a physician or other professional prior to beginning a stretching program. Medication, ice, heat, and other methods used prior to exercise is often a standard recommendation for these patients. It is, however, important to understand the risks and side effects of any treatment for pain before regular use. Even if a chronic medical condition makes the routine use of over-the-counter medication unsafe, alternatives are always available from a qualified health professional.

INCORPORATING STRETCHING INTO YOUR EXERCISE ROUTINE

It is important to remember that, despite the research that is available, the health benefits of stretching alone have not been clearly established. Combining flexibility exercises with other modes, such as aerobic workouts and strength training, will provide the maximum improvements in overall health. No matter how old or young, anyone can participate in such a program with proper guidance and adaptations.

While the effect is modest, stretching probably confers at least some protection against injury during exercise, especially when performed regularly over long periods of time. Supervision by a professional, at least initially, is important for many. Certainly supervised flexibility exercises are important for those with physical injury or deformities of bones, joints, skin, or muscle. These individuals will benefit from understanding what limitations their injuries place on their ability to stretch and how to work around them. A skilled physical or occupational therapist can assist in prescribing an appropriate exercise regimen, usually under the guidance of a physician.

Even when achieving optimal range of motion is not crucial, stretching is useful as a "warm-up" activity before strenuous exercise. Flexibility exercises at this time can actually improve the blood flow through muscles and help them to work more efficiently and with less discomfort. Dynamic stretches may be especially useful for this as they can increase the heart rate in anticipation of exercise. On the other hand, static stretches that will reduce the heart rate after vigorous exercise are often used as a "cool-down" technique. In studies reviewed by Drs. I. Shrier and K. Gossal, greater gains in range of motion around joints is seen when static exercises are performed routinely after more intensive aerobic exercise or strength training. They also find stretching to be useful for pain relief after intense workouts, especially when combined with heat or ice.

The ACSM recommends incorporating stretches into a workout routine at least three times per week. Five to seven times per week is preferable as the effects of stretching are temporary and more regular exercises produces the best results. Static and dynamic exercises may be used, but ACSM advises caution and supervision for certain static stretches in inexperienced stretchers. These include any straight-knee hamstring stretches, aggressive knee bending, and certain other advanced stretching techniques. No matter which, the motion should produce a gentle yet definite stretching sensation in a given muscle group. Static poses should be held for about fifteen seconds and repeated several times in order to bring about useful changes in range of motion. Holding for thirty seconds is probably safe and may produce results quicker, when needed. Regardless of the duration, the maneuver should never be overtly painful.

For those who have been relatively inactive and would like to start their exercise gradually, stretching activities such as yoga or Tai Chi seem to improve balance and coordination—especially during walking. These disciplines offer several other advantages, such as supervision by a trained and certified instructor. Such classes are also social opportunities and people tend to maintain exercise programs more easily over time when they look forward to seeing friends during activity. In fact, these exercise regimens seem to have positive effects on mood and self-image, especially when combined with time-honored techniques such as breathing exercises and meditation. Even in life threatening medical conditions, such as cancer, yoga shows some promise for maintaining positive outlook and a sense of peace while undergoing treatment.

Those who are left with questions about flexibility should not hesitate to contact a knowledgeable health care professional. To date, we can definitively state that stretching has already been shown to have positive effects on health and function, and likely in the future, we'll learn more about the risks and benefits of this important exercise mode.

SELECTED BIBLIOGRAPHY

Askling C, Lund H, Saartok T, and Thorstensson A. "Self-reported hamstring injuries in student-dancers." *Scandinavian Journal of Medicine & Science in Sports* 12 (2002): 230–235.

Cress ME et al. "Physical activity programs and behavior counseling in older adult populations—best practices statement." *Medicine & Science in Sports & Exercise* (2004): 1997–2003.

Dadebo B et al. "A survey of flexibility training protocols and hamstring strains in professional football clubs in England." *British Journal of Sports Medicine* 38 (2003): 388–394.

DiBenedetto M et al. "Effect of a gentle Iyengar yoga program on gait in the elderly: An exploratory study." *Archives of Physical Medicine and Rehabilitation* 86 (2005): 1830–1837.

Frankel JE et al. "Exercise in the elderly: Research and clinical practice [review]." *Clinics in Geriatric Medicine* 22 (2006): 239–256.

Li F, et al. "Exercise in the elderly: Research and clinical practice." *Medicine & Science in Sports & Exercise* (2004): 2046–2052.

Motl RW et al. "Depressive symptoms among older adults: Long-term reduction after a physical activity intervention." *Journal of Behavioral Medicine* 28 (2005): 385–394.

Roberts JM and Wilson K. "Effect of stretching duration on active and passive range of motion in the lower extremity." *British Journal of Sports Medicine* 33 (1999): 259–263.

Saal JS. "Flexibility training." In *Functional Rehabilitation of Sports and Musculoskeletal Injuries*, Kibler WB (ed.) (Aspen, CO: Aspen Publishers, 1998), 85–95.

Tsang W and Hui-Chan C. "Comparison of muscle torque, balance, and confidence in older Tai Chi and healthy adults." *Medicine & Science in Sports & Exercise* (2005): 280–289.

6

FUNCTIONAL TRAINING HEALTH BENEFITS

Jeffrey C. Ives and Betsy Keller

...many [athletes] who have been perfectly proportioned fall into the hands of trainers who develop them beyond measure, overloaded them with flesh and blood, and make them just the opposite.

Despite these disadvantages athletes assert that they wish to be strong, and that strength is the one thing worth the while. Ye gods! How are they strong? And of what use is their strength? Is it of use on the farm? Can the athlete dig, harvest, or accomplish more in agriculture? Is he more apt in war? Recall anew the verses of Euripides who thus glorifies the athlete: "Do we combat with the discus in hand? The enemy approaching, we recognize the foolishness of this preparation.
—Galenius, Claudius. "Exhortation to Study the Arts." ca AD 180. Translation by J Walsh published in *Medical Life*, v. 37, pp. 507–529, 1930.

What Galen saw in Greek athletes nearly 1,900 years ago is just as observable in athletes today, and surprisingly, in a typical user of any modern day fitness center. Galen, the cantankerous physician-philosopher whose ideas dominated medicine for over 1,500 years, knew that exercise for the main purpose of "being fit" without regard to real world function would take an athlete only so far in performance, and be of little benefit to carrying out normal activities of daily life. Nowadays, these observations apply directly to exercisers robotically going through the motions—more sets, more reps, more miles—without much regard to anything other than fitness. There is more to exercise training than fitness, however, and that is function. The aim of this chapter is to describe what is meant by function and how functional training differs from other exercise regimens. It should be noted that designing an effective functional training program can be more dimensional than a standard aerobic or muscle fitness program and may require an experienced exercise professional to assess needs and prescribe training methods, particularly for those with a high degree of dysfunction. For many others, though, improving function like carrying a 10 lb. bag of groceries or moving a garbage can safely from the house to the curb can be devised with some basic knowledge and a little creativity.

HISTORY OF FUNCTIONAL TRAINING

The Greek athletes during Galen's time were not the historical norm. Historical records reveal that functional training, albeit not called that, has predominated for literally thousands of years. Primarily reserved for soldiers and athletes, dedicated physical training was focused toward specific functional outcomes. The Roman military demanded that mental and tactical skills be used in conjunction with physical skills and so Roman soldiers spent hours engaging in physical exercises designed to support and improve their weapon use and tactical skills. During the Age of Chivalry knights wrestled, scaled walls, threw heavy stones, and fought their way through obstacles. Knights donned full armor, often weighing 40–60 lbs. or more, and did somersaults and vaults to train for the agility required on the battlefield. The gymnastics pommel horse apparatus is a modern-day adaptation of training devices knights used to improve strength and ability for mounting and dismounting horses during battle. Essentially, training for athletes and soldiers consisted of making the required activities more challenging. Weapons were made heavier, heights were made higher, ground was made unstable, and obstacles more imposing. Soldiers were sometimes told to stay away from physical activities that might train them apart from military skills. In his 1438 book, *The Royal Book of Jousting Horsemanship and Knightly Combat*, King of Portugal Dom Duarte cautioned knights against ball-throwing games because they might improperly train their fencing arm. Except for those privileged few over the course of history who have had the luxury of leisure time to exercise for beauty, healthful vitality, and moral character, it appears that nonfunctional physical training is a relatively modern phenomenon.

It is unclear when the term "functional training" came into use or by whom. It may have originated in the early to mid-1900s within the physical rehabilitation medical specialties. A review article about functional training appeared in a 1949 issue of *Physical Therapy Review*, so its use certainly predates that time. Today, the concept of functional training takes on a variety of names, including functional rehabilitation, functional exercise, work hardening, added purpose training, neuromuscular training, psychophysical training, sport-specific training, and combat training, among others. Occupational preparedness, which includes military and sport training, and physical rehabilitation are the two areas in which functional training is used most extensively.

Like their ancient predecessors, the military continues to refine functional training to bring combat readiness safely to their soldiers by training both the specific physiological capabilities and movement abilities needed for combat. Foot soldiers crawl under barbed wire and climb over walls and scuba divers strain to pull weights through the water. The military, athletes, and rehabilitation patients now use virtual reality simulations to enhance the functional training experience. Athletes and coaches know that simply being bigger and stronger can only improve performance to a point. Functional training takes the movement demands of a real game, like an off-balance jump, twist, and reach, to the exercise setting where the athlete must make these movements under intensely challenging situations. Physical and occupational therapists use functional training extensively in orthopedic and physical rehabilitation. It is more effective, for example, to have a hand surgery patient practice holding and controlling a heavy cast-iron fry pan rather than do straightforward hand grip exercises. This type of rehabilitation, sometimes called "added purpose training," develops muscle strength in conjunction with the coordination necessary for daily life activities. In addition, adding purpose to the training provides motivation to a wearisome rehabilitation program, not to mention those in a monotonous fitness program.

Functional training concepts are gradually making their way from the rehabilitation and athletic settings to fitness centers for use by relatively healthy adults. The application of these concepts, however, is not often straightforward. The next section describes in more detail the use of functional training for relatively healthy adult populations who are training to improve wellness and performance in activities of daily living, decrease the risks of injury and falls, and prevent decline in function later in life.

WHAT MAKES TRAINING FUNCTIONAL?

Functional training for relatively healthy adults has become a buzzword applied to training modes that have certain characteristics. These characteristics include posture and balance, agility, "core" training, free form resistance training (e.g., medicine balls and elastic bands), martial arts (e.g., Tai Chi, yoga), and choreographed calisthenics. None of these characteristics, however, makes an exercise program functional. It is the purpose of exercise, not the type of exercise, which distinguishes functional training. Without an intentional purpose directed at improving the quality of movement, functional training is simply training.

Functional training is broadly defined as training to improve real-world physical performance, otherwise known as activities of daily living. These activities of daily living (ADLs) are just that; they are the things people do on a daily or weekly basis. Some activities are home-based, like getting out of bed, bathing, gardening, walking up and down stairs, cooking, lugging grocery bags, carrying children, and housework. Some activities predominate at work, such as computer use, truck driving, tool and machine use, assembly work, firefighting and rescue, and any number of other occupational tasks. Other activities are specific to hobbies or leisure time, like sports and games. People often struggle to do these activities effectively and without pain, but prior injury or illness, overuse and maladaption to chronic use, deconditioning, or biological degeneration due to aging, may make that difficult. Functional training aims at improving either general movement qualities or specific movement skills so that these movements become easier, freer, more adaptable, and more comfortable when done in their real-life context.

The counterpart to functional training, functional health, is one's capability to participate effectively in wide-ranging activities of daily living, regardless of any underlying pathology or mental or physical illness. An adaptable motor system characterizes functional health, enabling a diverse repertoire of movements that permits individuals to engage in physical activities that are both necessary and desirable components of a rich and fulfilling life. The purpose of functional training is foremost to help one develop this repertoire to enable effective movements with confidence and without discomfort during normal daily activities at home, work, and play.

This objective of functional training differs from that of conventional exercise regimens. The purpose of conventional cardiovascular and muscle fitness training is to enhance the basic physiological workings of the body, like increasing cardiac output, boosting cellular metabolism, and hypertrophying muscle tissue. Enhanced physiological systems are certainly a good thing—improving overall health and lowering disease risk—but this does not mean an automatic improvement to function efficiently and relatively pain-free throughout normal activities of daily life. The relationships among physiological mechanisms and real-life performance can be better understood by looking at the Model of Disablement, a framework sanctioned by the World Health Organization to track the progression from disease to disability:

Pathology >> Impairment >> Functional Limitation >> Disability

Pathology, the underlying disease or physiological abnormality, contributes to *impairment* in how tissues or systems operate. These systems may be physiological or psychological. Impairment contributes to *functional limitation*, which is difficulty in performing ADLs. If functional limitation disrupts ability to function in society, it becomes a *disability*. For example, consider that tissue degeneration of arthritis (pathology) leads to joint pain, weakness, and loss of range of motion (impairment). These impairment may lead to difficulty in opening jars and cans (functional limitation), which may further lead to an inability to function independently in one's own kitchen (disability). Figure 6.1 illustrates that this model is not a simple continuum; for the progression from pathology to disability is an interaction of multiple factors, and can even progress backward, as in the case of functional limitations and disabilities that lead to inactivity and hypokinetic diseases. Hypokinetic diseases, for example atherosclerosis and diabetes, are diseases caused to some extent by a lack of physical activity. The same impairment may result in a functional limitation in one person, a different limitation in another person, and no impairment in still another. Progression is linked to the extent of the impairment, the number of other impairments and associated problems, psychosocial factors, strategies one uses to adapt to dysfunction, and a host of genetic and acquired risk factors that can predispose one to more serious consequences.

Figure 6.1
The Model of Disablement Illustrates the Progression of Disease
to Disability

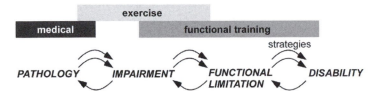

Progression along the continuum is mostly left to right, but not always. It is not
always direct as indicated by the curved arrows. Numerous risk factors
influence if and how one level progresses to the next. Key risk factors are:
-Demographic (e.g., age, socioeconomic status, education)
-Physiological (e.g., body size, diet, gender)
-Environmental (e.g., housing, climate, occupation)
-Co-morbidities (e.g., hypertension, diabetes, obesity)

Notice the overlap among the medical, exercise, and functional training
interventions, but that functional training targets a broader scope than other
methods. An important target for functional training is the development of
effective strategies to prevent functional limitations from becoming disabilities.

The goal of functional training, ultimately, is to stop impairments from
becoming functional limitations and stop functional impairments from
becoming disabilities. Improving functional health may increase one's
activity level and psychological status, thereby having a positive effect
on impairments and pathologies.

Source: Jeffrey C. Ives.

The traditional medical and exercise approach addresses problems primarily at the pathological and impairment level, which potentially can have a positive effect on functional limitations and disability. This is certainly the right approach in many instances, but the complexity of disablement model means that even if a pathology or impairment restores to normal, the functional limitations and disability may remain. What is deemed normal or acceptable by rehabilitative standards may still include a tolerance of asymmetric movement or restricted joint motion that may be exacerbated with normal use or with a traditional exercise program. Likewise, often times the pathology or impairment cannot be reversed, forcing individuals to learn to live with the disabling consequences of chronic health problems. The functional training approach is designed to address functional limitations, and to a lesser extent, disability, thereby improving functional health.

FUNCTIONAL TRAINING FOR FUNCTIONAL HEALTH

There are two categories of health issues, therapeutic and preventative, that can benefit from functional training. *Therapeutic* health issues are functional limitations brought about by known health problems, such as osteoarthritis and low back pain. The therapeutic label should not be misunderstood to mean that the health issues are so bad as to require medical attention. Many lingering health problems remain after even successful medical interventions or are not severe enough for individuals to believe medical intervention is necessary (e.g., sprained ankle, chronic low back discomfort). *Preventive* health issues include strategies to maximize current performance and minimize risks of future functional limitations. In this category are generally healthy individuals training for vocational readiness (work hardening and prehabilitation training), sport-specific training including that for the weekend athlete, and those trying to prevent later functional decline, such as with mobility and fall prevention for older adults. There is considerable overlap between therapeutic and preventative functional training, as a program can address both current limitations and prevention of further decline in function. This is especially true in older adults, who often need to address current health issues and train to prevent disabling problems like falls. This situation is illustrated in the case study presented at the end of the chapter.

Therapeutic: Musculoskeletal and Other Chronic Health Problems

Therapeutic functional training may improve physical function and reduce discomfort, even in the face of an ongoing disease process or damaged tissues that make movement difficult. For example, arthritis, multiple sclerosis, old tissue damage from injury or disease, cardiovascular disease, and a large number of other chronic health problems result in painful and dysfunctional movement patterns that cascade into more dysfunction and pain. Even minor problems considered by many to be simply bothersome or just a part of normal aging, such as muscle aches, restricted joint range of motion, and muscle weakness, may contribute to the cascade of dysfunction and pain. Many of these health problems are found in the elderly, but by no means are middle aged and younger adults invulnerable. In fact, it is likely that most adult members of fitness centers exercise to overcome nagging musculoskeletal problems and similar problems run rampant in both blue and white collar occupational settings.

A large number of scientific studies have reported successful functional training outcomes. Factory workers have overcome chronic neck and shoulder musculoskeletal pain, young and middle-aged individuals have recovered from low back pain and learned to manage joint pain from prior injury. Knee and ankle injury prevalence have been reduced in young athletes, carpal tunnel syndrome and other repetitive strain injuries alleviated in office and factory workers, and better functioning in daily activities have been reported in sufferers of osteoarthritis and multiple sclerosis. Functional training has helped individuals with very poor exercise capacity due to cardiopulmonary problems to overcome some of their disability through improved functional strength and efficiency of movement. Seemingly, an impressive result for sure, but functional training is no cure all. It has also proven ineffective in many instances where, for example, degenerative or damaged joint architecture precluded normal joint range of motion.

Preventative: Fall Prevention and Activities of Daily Living

Numerous reports over the past twenty years generally indicate that fall prevention programs are effective in relatively healthy elders and frail and institutionalized elders suffering from physical and mental impairments. Often these programs include multiple strategies alongside functional exercise, like reducing psychotropic drug doses, safety education, and reduction of environmental risk factors. In recent years there have been several "systematic reviews" that summarized scientific studies on functional training. These reviews indicate that functional exercise programs improve performance on functional laboratory tests (e.g., walking speed, grip strength, rising out of a chair), but real-world performance like reducing the number of falls has been difficult to measure. Even Tai Chi, widely popularized over the past fifteen years in part due to a few studies that showed large benefits for improving elderly mobility, has not shown to produce consistently positive effects. Part of the problem, as concluded by researchers like Verhagen and her colleagues at the Erasmus Medical Center in Rotterdam, is simply that many of these scientific studies do not sufficiently tease out the complexities that contribute to functional declines.[1] Researchers do agree that effective exercise training programs tend to be multimodal (e.g., strength and balance and gait training) and are targeted toward individual problems. The success of a functional training program hinges solely on the carry-over of training improvements to benefit real-life activities.

If there is one thing that has emerged from the science, it is that there is a great deal of individual variation in how one responds to training and how training adaptations transfer to the real world. Some individuals show remarkable improvements whereas others doing the same training program show none. This stands in contrast to standard fitness programs in which the vast majority of participants who engage in the same exercise mode of sufficient intensity realize some physiological improvements. This illustrates that most scientific studies of functional training lack the essential ingredient of providing individual-based training prescriptions. Prominent geriatric exercise physiologist, Jack Rejeski, PhD, and his fellow scientists at Wake Forest University noted that it is difficult to prescribe a standardized functional training program and asserted that the large role sociocultural factors play in influencing real-world performance is often overlooked.[2] These scientists believe that functional training programs must, within the actual context of training, address beliefs and symptoms that influence how and if one performs physical tasks. For instance, exercise training in a comfortable and controlled environment may be ineffective in helping improve stair climbing in a frenzied workplace because one's confidence and self-image in the face of judgmental and impatient coworkers are critical in determining even if stair climbing will be attempted.

The efficacy of functional training in younger, healthy people to prevent decline later in life remains to be determined. The key issue is if the functional training program targets the right combination of factors that lead to a decline in function. For example, can mobility and balance training in a middle-aged adult help prevent falls and a decline in gait speed and improve stair climbing in old age? We do know that high intensity strength training in middle-aged persons can improve functional laboratory tasks like 10-meter walking speed and balance measurements, but will this carry over to a reduction in falls twenty years later? At this time it is speculative to suggest that it will, however it is likely that a well-conceived regimen practiced throughout life will reduce the loss of function later in life.

FUNCTIONAL HEALTH EVALUATION

Effective functional training requires careful client evaluation and observation to determine the individual needs of the client, the goals of the functional training program, and the exercise techniques to accomplish those goals. Unfortunately, there is no one-size-fits-all or gold standard of testing because the functional impairments and needs vary widely across individuals and populations. Thus, ingredients for an effective functional training program, whether therapeutic or preventative, should satisfy the following criteria to improve functional health:

- Identify individual needs
- Application to real-world physical challenges
- Appropriate for current level of physical function
- Systematic increase in physical challenge
- Accessible for user in the environment in which the user is most likely to function

These criteria are discussed further in this section and throughout the remainder of the chapter.

Individual Needs

Identification of individual needs begins with a functional health evaluation. The majority of functional health evaluation protocols (also called functional performance evaluation) have been developed and used for unhealthy persons (physical rehabilitation and frail elders) and for specific vocational settings, and may not work well for relatively healthy adults. Nevertheless, by looking at the functional health evaluation process we can gather general strategies for use in relatively healthy populations.

Functional health evaluation aims at understanding what movements and tasks are dysfunctional, why that movement is dysfunctional, how the individual deals with it, and finally, the goals of the individual. Typically, this includes a subjective assessment of the client based on questionnaires, medical history, and quality of life (what, how, and why of client's current state); an objective assessment of the client based on functional performance tests (what can/can't client do?); and finally, interpretation of subjective and objective information to evaluate degree of limitation and identification of goals.

Subjective Assessment via Questionnaires

Numerous questionnaires have been developed to identify functional limitations or level of discomfort associated with ADLs. Questionnaires may be general surveys of health-related quality of life, such as the Medical Outcomes 36-Item Short Form Health Survey (SF-36; Figure 6.2), but most focus on identifying problem areas in individuals with known health issues, such as the Oswestry Low Back Pain Questionnaire and the Musculoskeletal Function Assessment. Good questionnaires help identify what the problems are and why the problems exist. It is often the case that functional problems arise from medical issues but then persist and spiral downward because of psychosocial issues like fear and avoidance, pain, poor self-esteem, missing social networks, and so forth. Questionnaires should also inquire about how individuals deal with dysfunction and their general beliefs about their symptoms and functional status. There are but a handful of questionnaires that are reliable and valid, and so the selection, use, and interpretation of the questionnaires is best left to experienced professionals, such as exercise physiologists or physical therapists who are experienced in functional performance evaluation and functional exercise programming.

Objective Assessment via Functional Performance Evaluation

Functional performance tests use standardized and objective criteria to measure aspects of performance to assess functional decline, predict later disability, and provide targets for intervention. Tests vary from single tasks to examine specific movement limitations in activities of daily living (e.g., rising out of a chair), to batteries of multiple tests designed to assess a range of functional, cognitive, and physical performance capabilities. Some researchers have developed what they consider single all-in-one tests, like the lateral mobility test shown in Figure 6.3. Performance evaluation on most tests is a combination of a quantifiable rating scale and a subjective visual determination of movement quality, like symmetry, steadiness, and coordination.

Test batteries typically center on a specific theme, such as vocational skills (both healthy and unhealthy workers), sport-related skills (athletes), or home-based activities of daily living (for elders and impaired adults). Popular functional test batteries for home-based activities include the Continuous-Scale Physical Functional Performance[3] and the Physical Performance Test.[4] These

Figure 6.2
The SF-36 Health Survey

INSTRUCTIONS: This set of questions asks for your views about your health. This information will help keep track of how you feel and how well you are able to do your usual activities. Answer every question by marking the answer as indicated. If you are unsure about how to answer a question please give the best answer you can.	

1. In general, would you say your health is: (Please tick **one** box.)

Excellent	☐
Very Good	☐
Good	☐
Fair	☐
Poor	☐

2. Compared to one year ago, how would you rate your health in general now? (Please tick **one** box.)

Much better than one year ago	☐
Somewhat better now than one year ago	☐
About the same as one year ago	☐
Somewhat worse now than one year ago	☐
Much worse now than one year ago	☐

3. The following questions are about activities you might do during a typical day. Does your health now limit you in these activities? If so, how much? **(Please circle one number on each line.)**

	Activities	Yes, Limited A Lot	Yes, Limited A Little	Not Limited At All
3(a)	**Vigorous activities**, such as running, lifting heavy objects, participating in strenuous sports	1	2	3
3(b)	**Moderate activities**, such as moving a table, pushing a vacuum cleaner, bowling, or playing golf	1	2	3
3(c)	Lifting or carrying groceries	1	2	3
3(d)	Climbing **several** flights of stairs	1	2	3
3(e)	Climbing **one** flight of stairs	1	2	3
3(f)	Bending, kneeling, or stooping	1	2	3
3(g)	Waling **more than a mile**	1	2	3
3(h)	Walking **several blocks**	1	2	3
3(i)	Walking **one block**	1	2	3
3(j)	Bathing or dressing yourself	1	2	3

4. During the past 4 weeks, have you had any of the following problems with your work or other regular daily activities as a result of your physical health? **(Please circle one number on each line.)**

		Yes	No
4(a)	Cut down on the **amount of time** you spent on work or other activities	1	2
4(b)	Accomplished less than you would like	1	2
4(c)	Were **limited** in the **kind** of work or other activities	1	2
4(d)	Had **difficulty** performing the work or other activities (for example, it took extra effort)	1	2

5. During the past 4 weeks, have you had any of the following problems with your work or other regular daily activities as a result of any emotional problems (e.g. feeling depressed or anxious)? **(Please circle one number on each line.)**

		Yes	No
5(a)	Cut down on the **amount of time** you spent on work or other activities	1	2
5(b)	Accomplished less than you would like	1	2
5(c)	Didn't do work or other activities as **carefully** as usual	1	2

Figure 6.2
(*continued*)

6.	During the <u>past 4 weeks</u>, to what extent has your physical health or emotional problems interfered with your normal social activities with family, friends, neighbours, or groups? (Please tick **one** box.)	
	Not at all ☐	
	Slightly ☐	
	Moderately ☐	
	Quite a bit ☐	
	Extremely ☐	

7.	How much <u>physical</u> pain have you had during the <u>past 4 weeks</u>? (Please tick **one** box.)
	None ☐
	Very mild ☐
	Mild ☐
	Moderate ☐
	Severe ☐
	Very Severe ☐

8.	During the <u>past 4 weeks</u>, how much did <u>pain</u> interfere with your normal work (including both work outside the home and housework)? (Please tick **one** box.)
	Not at all ☐
	A little bit ☐
	Moderately ☐
	Quite a bit ☐
	Extremely ☐

9. These questions are about how you feel and how things have been with you <u>during the past 4 weeks</u>. Please give the one answer that is closest to the way you have been feeling for each item.

(Please circle one number on each line.)	All of the Time	Most of the Time	A Good Bit of the Time	Some of the Time	A Little of the Time	None of the Time
9(a) Did you feel full of life?	1	2	3	4	5	6
9(b) Have you been a very nervous person?	1	2	3	4	5	6
9(c) Have you felt so down in the dumps that nothing could cheer you up?	1	2	3	4	5	6
9(d) Have you felt calm and peaceful?	1	2	3	4	5	6
9(e) Did you have a lot of energy?	1	2	3	4	5	6
9(f) Have you felt downhearted and blue?	1	2	3	4	5	6
9(g) Did you feel worn out?	1	2	3	4	5	6
9(h) Have you been a happy person?	1	2	3	4	5	6
9(i) Did you feel tired?	1	2	3	4	5	6

10.	During the <u>past 4 weeks</u>, how much of the time has your <u>physical health or emotional problems</u> interfered with your social activities (like visiting with friends, relatives etc.) (Please tick **one** box.)
	All of the time ☐
	Most of the time ☐
	Some of the time ☐
	A little of the time ☐
	None of the time ☐

11. How TRUE or FALSE is <u>each</u> of the following statements for you?

(Please circle one number on each line.)	Definitely True	Mostly True	Donít Know	Mostly False	Definitely False
11(a) I seem to get sick a little easier than other people	1	2	3	4	5
11(b) I am as healthy as anybody I know	1	2	3	4	5
11(c) I expect my health to get worse	1	2	3	4	5
11(d) My health is excellent	1	2	3	4	5

Thank You!

Source: Ware JE, Kosinski M, Dewey JE. How to Score Version 2 of the SF-36® Health Survey. Lincoln, RI: QualityMetric Incorporated, 2000. SF-36v2™ Health Survey 1996, 2000 by QualityMetric Incorporated. All Rights Reserved. SF-36v2™ is a trademark of QualityMetric.

Figure 6.3
Lateral Mobility Functional Assessment

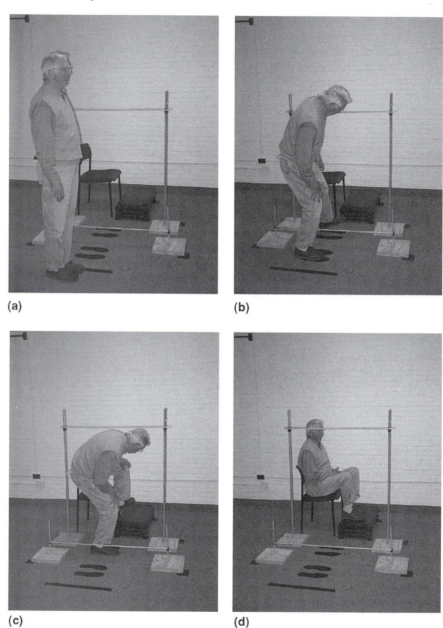

(a)   (b)

(c)   (d)

This simple test requires single leg strength and balance, trunk stability, leg and truck flexibility, and sensory awareness.

Source: Reprinted, with permission, from A.P. Marsh, W.J. Rejeski, S.L. Hutton, C.L. Brown, E. Ip, and J.M. Guralnik, "Development of a Lateral Mobility Task to Identify Individuals at Risk for Mobility Disability and Functional Decline," *Journal of Aging and Physical Activity* 13 (4): (2005).

test batteries include items such as timed stair walking, picking up a penny, simulated eating, writing a sentence, pouring a gallon jug of liquid, putting on a jacket, and carrying weights to mimic a grocery or laundry bag. In addition to assessing specific skills, careful interpretation of the test results enables the practitioner to determine potential underlying causes of the functional limitations, such as loss of range of motion or muscle weakness. Other test batteries are less task-specific, instead focusing on general function, like the Performance Oriented Mobility Assessment[5] that focuses on balance and gait. The most common balance test is timed one-leg standing with eyes open and eyes closed, but other tests include standing balance while being nudged and the ability to turn 360 degrees without staggering. Gait is assessed for speed, steadiness, and symmetry of left and right step length. Balance and gait are often assessed together with heel-to-toe line walking (or on a balance beam) and the timed sit-to-stand-to-walk test. In the latter, persons are evaluated on steadiness in rising out of a chair without using their arms, steadiness upon standing and transitioning to walking, ability to walk and turn around, and ability to control descent back into a sitting position.

Functional Assessment of Relatively Healthy Adults

Functional performance assessment for relatively healthy middle-aged adults and high-functioning elders is scarce, but there have been some attempts to provide guidelines in testing these individuals based on modifications to functional training assessments for frail and unhealthy adults. Because low back pain is such a common condition among adults who consider themselves otherwise healthy, it is appropriate to assess risk factors for low back pain.

Initial health screening begins with a medical history and a general assessment of the client's health-related quality of life, such as the SF-36. The SF-36 questionnaire measures eight dimensions from physical functioning and bodily pain to mental health and social functioning. Results from the initial screening may indicate the need for functional performance testing, but even if not, administering a limited number of general functional performance tests that have a sound basis for prediction of later functional limitations is prudent. The functional performance test batteries (Figure 6.4) have reasonable test reliability, plausible validity to predict later disability, and are able to discriminate between higher functioning and moderate functioning individuals, and older versus younger people. These tests focus on strength of the arms and legs, postural control, balance, and gait. They are described here with criterion values purposely omitted, only to help the reader understand the nature of the tests, because the actual testing and interpretation of the results requires some level of knowledge. Careful observation of movement quality during test performance is also essential. Stuart McGill, PhD, a spine biomechanist at the University of Waterloo and author of what may be the evidence-based bible of low back function, *Low Back Disorders; Evidence-Based Prevention and Rehabilitation*, has devised several low back screening tests. One of his simpler

Figure 6.4
Functional Test Batteries

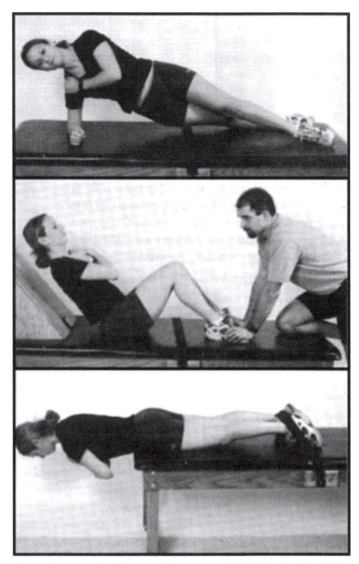

Source: Reprinted, with permission, from S. McGill, *Low Back Disorders: Evidence-based Prevention and Rehabilitation*, 2nd ed. (Champaign, IL: Human Kinetics, 2007), 225–226.

tests, also listed with reference values, again, is for informational purposes only.

In summary, functional testing for unhealthy adults, and relatively healthy or frail older adults, requires knowledge and familiarity with functional assessment to identify the appropriate testing methods, conduct the tests reliably and safely, and interpret the tests correctly. Functional health testing for healthy middle aged and highly functioning older adults is still in the developmental stage, but some gait, posture, and muscle function tests hold promise in providing guidelines for functional exercise prescription.

EXERCISE PRESCRIPTION FOR FUNCTIONAL TRAINING

Numerous exercise regimens have been passed on as functional training, but exercise mode is only important if it satisfies a functional purpose. Training to improve functional task outcomes requires understanding of the movements, environments, and circumstances in which activities are performed. Functional training brings the situational needs and constraints of the actual activity into the training environment (*application to real-world physical challenges*) and creates situations where there can be both training overload and exaggerated situational needs and constraints (*appropriate for current level of physical function; systematic increase in physical challenge*). Figure 6.5 illustrates that an individual's psychological and physiological make-up interacts with the environment and task demands, from which purposeful functional movement is developed. Only by incorporating environmental situations and task demands into the training program can training be considered truly functional.

Taken collectively, functional training for fall prevention, general mobility, specific ADLs can be addressed by basic fitness, functional mobility challenge training, and self-efficacy improvement. Functional training aimed at overcoming specific musculoskeletal and chronic health problems requires additional steps to train movement patterns that alleviate discomfort and avoid making the problem worse. This step requires more than can be covered here and so we will focus on the three basic steps.

Fall Prevention, General Mobility, Specific ADLs

First addressed are the basic components of fitness (strength, aerobic, flexibility), particularly in frail older adults and others who are highly deconditioned. The specific fitness demands of the task (see Figure 6.5) are emphasized while also taking into consideration impairments shown to be strongly associated with later functional declines. Leg and arm strength are important components of many tasks; a lack of strength is implicated in many functional declines and thus can be a starting point for many functional training programs. General mobility and movement training is then added, with increasing level of challenge, variability, and uncertainty to focus on functional needs. The purpose of this functional "mobility challenge" training is to enhance the

Figure 6.5
Systems Approach to Functional Training

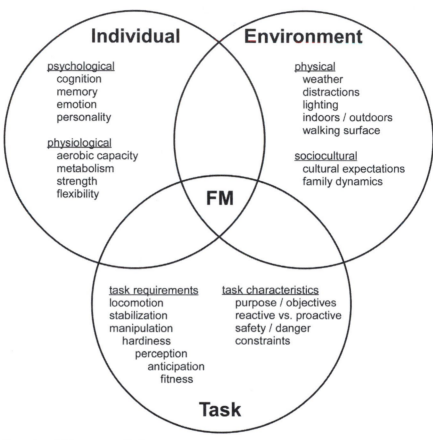

Functional Movement (FM) is produced by an individual in the context of various environmental and task circumstances and based on the individual's physiological and psychological makeup. Functional training takes into account the capabilities of the individual and designed with the task and environmental characteristics in mind.

Source: Jeffrey C. Ives.

response to balance threats that are necessary for real-life environments, develop adaptable and responsive postural control strategies, improve movement ease and effectiveness, and develop self-efficacy. The strategies devised in the mobility challenge training draw upon the environmental and task issues illustrated in Figure 6.5 and the functional impairments revealed through testing. Examples include walking over obstacles and on unstable or slippery surfaces, asymmetric load carrying while pivoting, "speed" walking against the flow of foot traffic, reduced lighting, dual task challenges like engaging in a conversation while walking, reaching and stretching while walking, and combinations of the above. These first two tiers of the framework address the multiple bio-logical and functional problems associated with falls and mobility problems.

Development of self-efficacy is often ignored. It should be incorporated into the entire functional training package to facilitate transfer of the training to real life circumstances and the sociocultural environment. Self-efficacy, or one's belief in their competence to perform or carry out tasks, is an important contributor to functional health and self-regulation of health behaviors like adherence to training. Understanding the self-efficacy beliefs of individual clients requires purposeful inquiry and careful observation and is a vital aspect of assessing the functional training needs in elders and those with low back pain and other chronic health problems. Training for self-efficacy may include educational sessions or just a careful progression of exercise challenges that develop a sense of mastery and empowerment in the clients.

Notes on Posture and Balance Training

Posture and balance training are rightly important components of many functional training programs, but often misunderstood and misapplied. Postu-ral control mechanisms that control posture (orientation of body) and balance (stability of body) are part of an unseen foundation that underpins every movement we make. While we place attention on a movement or movement outcome, such as reaching into a cupboard, our body undergoes a complex chain of postural movements without us knowing about it. Even before reach-ing into the cupboard our leg and trunk muscles stiffen in just the right manner to stabilize our spine and pelvis, our neck muscles orient our head, and our feet press down to prevent us from toppling over—all of this happening auto-matically while our attention is focused on a jar of honey on the top shelf. If we reach a bit to the left, or a little higher, if the floor is slippery, or if the jar is teetering precariously, then our postural responses change to match the circumstances. It is only when postural control mechanisms fail that we begin to notice them.

Some postural control mechanisms are innate to all of us, but by adulthood we have integrated these mechanisms into our own learned postural responses that become automatic. Our brain learns postural control by trial and error, taking into account our own body's physiological (e.g., muscle strength, reaction time, pain) and psychological factors (e.g., anxiety and self-efficacy beliefs) and habitual movements. Sometimes we learn poor postural habits, as in the case of holding our arms and shoulders at odd angles during hours of typing or holding an extreme pelvic tilt during prolonged sitting.

A variety of different balance training exercises appear to be effective in training better automatic postural control, but like most functional training methods, the techniques are specific to the desired movement outcome and the individual's psychological and physiological characteristics. For example, jumping and landing training that emphasizes biomechanically stable land-ings can help prevent some knee and ankle injuries, but computerized balance training may not. Some types of back exercises—with and without psychosocial interventions—have been successful in reducing low back pain, as have some mental imagery training programs. Movement training and postural awareness approaches can be successful in helping office workers alter their movements and thereby reduce repetitive strain injuries to the wrists and shoulders, but sitting on a Swiss ball probably will not. The important similarity among successful posture and balance techniques is inclusion of training that mimics actual task demands and environmental challenges.

What about functional training for healthy adults with no functional limitations? Can nonspecific functional training prevent widespread functional decline in later years? The current trend in posture and balance training for healthy adults, such as wobble board balance exercises, Swiss ball training, and low intensity martial arts, certainly aims in this direction. However, it is unlikely that nonspecific training will prevent multiple potential deficits. Generic postural training may enhance some balance mechanisms that contribute to some functional limitations. In addition, there is evidence that a challenging balance program may help maintain some sensory-motor systems (e.g., vestibulo-motor) and slow the development of impairments. To some extent, fitness training aimed at overcoming impairments (e.g., strength, stamina, flexibility, agility) can include functional challenges. In this way, fitness becomes integrated with motor skills and postural control and thus, more useful. Even if functional improvement is secondary to fitness training, it is still best to target the functional training toward prevalent functional health problems that are likely to arise. These prevalent health issues include fall prevention and limitations arising from back and shoulder musculoskeletal problems. These problems, like bursitis and shoulder pain, contribute to painful lifting and reaching and negatively affect anything from keyboard entry and assembly line work to carrying children.

TOOLS, EQUIPMENT, AND MODES OF TRAINING

Designing a functional training program requires expertise, creativity, and a trial and error attitude. High-tech equipment and instructor enthusiasm cannot take the place of a rational and assessment-driven training program designed to meet the functional health needs of an individual (*accessible for user in the environment in which the user is most likely to function*). Technologically advanced equipment used in research is now making its way into general use, including computerized postural control trainers, harness-supported gait trainers, and perturbation platforms. The market is bursting with elastic band gizmos, wobble board widgets, and core stabilization gadgets. None of these are more successful than low tech approaches. Indeed, some of the most successful interventions have been decidedly low or no tech, taking advantage of items around the house or office. Chairs, stairs, sticks, stools, and foam pads are common tools that can be used.

In a similar manner, there is no preferred mode, alone or in combination with other techniques, of training. Tai Chi may help prevent falls in some elders, strength training may be a better solution for others, and gait challenge training better for someone else. Body awareness and posture training has been shown to help workers overcome neck and shoulder pain at work, but then, so has relaxation training and some forms of strength training. In some workers these interventions have had no success. Unfortunately, even a rational and evidenced-based functional training program may end up being ineffective. If so, it is necessary to approach the problem from a different perspective and try again with the understanding that there is no magic bullet exercise.

PRECAUTIONS

Functional training is no different from other physical training methods in the need for proper screening of individuals to ensure their health for exercise. Though some functional training programs are not strenuous, others require high intensity cardiovascular and strength training. Unlike traditional training, functional training may pose balance and falling threats, and thereby requires direct supervision. Even some of the simplest challenges like one-leg standing and stepping over obstacles can be physically and mentally frustrating and pose a falling threat. Progression in functional training is calculated and intentional, and occurs only when the client has mastered each level. Matching training techniques and level of challenge to the abilities of the client is imperative.

FUTURE CONSIDERATIONS

Functional training holds a great deal of promise, indeed we see that much of the exercise training in the future will be aimed at improving functional health. Better ways of functional assessment are continually being developed and these assessment methods will enable more precise functional exercise prescriptions. Though functional exercise programs require no high-tech approaches, the flood of technological advancements will continue to find their way into functional exercise. Exercise equipment will be touted as "functional" and will include things such as treadmills that provide balance challenges and obstacle avoidance, strength training equipment with perturbations and asymmetric loading, and computerized balance and postural control trainers. Virtual reality technology will enable one to exercise while interacting within virtual environments, creating functional scenarios. Virtual reality technology, used extensively in the military and aeronautics, is just a few years away from being commonplace. Computer games have already joined the realm of functional, in which players must perform actual physical actions to produce the same simulated action on screen. These most recent attempts to integrate technology to positively impact physical function confirms that functional training is in and will stay in. After all, it has been around for thousands of years.

REFERENCES

1. Verhagen, A., Immink, M., van der Meulen, A., Bierma-Zeinstra, S. "The efficacy of Tai Chi Chuan in older adults: a systematic review." *Family Practice* 21 (2004): 107–113.

2. Rejeski, W., Brawley, L. "Functional health: Innovations in research on physical activity with older adults." *Medicine and Science in Sports and Exercise* 38 (2006): 93–99.

3. Cress, M., Buchner, D., Questad, K., Esselman, P., deLateur, B., Schwartz, R. "Continuous-scale physical functional performance in healthy older adults: A validation study." *Archives of Physical Medicine and Rehabilitation* 77 (1996): 1243–1250.

4. Reuben, D., Siu, A. "An objective measure of physical function of elderly outpatients. The Physical Performance Test." *Journal of the American Geriatrics Society* 38 (1990): 1105–1112.

5. Tinetti, M. "Performance-oriented assessment of mobility problems in elderly patients." *Journal of the American Geriatrics Society* 34 (1986): 119–126.

7

SPORT–SPECIFIC HEALTH BENEFITS

Jennifer Baima and William Mosi Jones

Sports participation offers an exciting format for vigorous exercise. A study of Harvard alumni over the years from 1962 to 1985 looked at the effect of vigorous physical activity on mortality. In this study of 10,000 men, initiating or continuing with sports participation resulted in an over 20 percent lower risk of death than not performing moderately vigorous physical activity. An interesting phenomenon became apparent when comparing the men in this study who had been collegiate athletes with those who had not participated in college sports. Surprisingly, both groups derived the same benefit of lower mortality.[1]

People who exercise every week have a healthier coronary risk factor profile. This benefit lasts for only two weeks if you stop exercising! Two studies evaluated former athletes and their current risk for coronary heart disease.[2,3] Contemporary sports participation rather than prior sports participation resulted in the observed cardiovascular benefit. Prior athleticism did not matter. This is great news for older adults looking to begin a new sport for exercise.

Exercise physiologists have used cardiac and pulmonary parameters to measure the energy expended during physical activity. In order to compare relative energy of different physical activities, the metabolic equivalent (MET) was developed. The energy that the body requires for one minute of sitting is one MET. This value rises with increased physical activity[4,5] (Table 7.1). It is sometimes difficult to assign METs to each sport as there is great complexity among the activities required during a given sport. This is due to variability of activity level intensity within a sport, the rules of the sport, and level of competition.

During a football game, a player may be accelerating, decelerating, jumping, pivoting, reaching, catching, colliding, or even throwing. There will be time spent in warm-up activities and resting on the sideline. Nearly four full-length basketball courts could fit on a football field. However, both sports involve periods of prolonged sprinting. A baseball or softball player does not run during every play as in football and basketball. He spends most of the inning

Table 7.1
Energy Requirements for Level of Activity

Activity Level	Energy Requirement
Light	<3.0 METs or <4 kcal/min
Moderate	3.0–6.0 METs or 4–7 kcal/min
Vigorous	>6.0 METs or >7 kcal/min

Source: Modified from Ref. 5.

his team is "at bat" in the dugout. Golfers may carry their clubs or hire a caddy. Tennis players can compete alone or in pairs. Different muscles are utilized for sculling as compared to kayaking, yet both may be considered rowing sports. Walking requires different energy utilization than competing in a triathlon.

As a result, the American College of Sports Medicine (ACSM) developed another method of classifying aerobic exercise into three groups based on activity demands.[4,6] Group I activities provide a consistent intensity and energy expenditure that are not dependent on the participant's skill level. These would include activities such as walking, cycling, jogging, and simulated stair climbing. With Group II activities, the rate of energy expenditure will vary greatly depending on the person's performance ability. With higher skill levels, a person can work harder and longer and consequently burn more calories. Activities in this category would include aerobic dancing, bench stepping, hiking, swimming, and water aerobics. The Group III activities, such as basketball, racquet sports, and volleyball are highly variable in terms of energy expenditure due to the performance demands of the activity.

The overall benefits of regular exercise include improved strength and endurance, healthier bones and muscles, weight reduction or control, anxiety reduction, increased self-esteem, and better blood pressure and cholesterol levels. The ACSM endorses aerobic exercise performed three to five days a week for twenty to sixty minutes, at an intensity that achieves 55 to 90 percent of the maximum heart rate and 40 to 85 percent of the maximum oxygen uptake reserve.[7] In place of one twenty- to sixty-minute session on a given day, the recommendations state that two to six ten-minute periods of aerobic activity throughout the day can be used to fulfill the requirements for the amount of exercise. Resistance training and flexibility training should also be incorporated in to the exercise routine. In calories, one should expend 150 to 400 kilocalories a day to obtain the desired health benefits of exercise. Sports such as bowling and shuffle board may not expend enough calories to result in the desired health benefit (Table 7.2).

It is important to remember that not all sports provide the same level of health benefit and certain sports confer additional benefits other than cardiovascular fitness. The addition of sports to your exercise routine can lead to increased consistency of participation as well as decreased overuse injury.

Table 7.2
Examples of Common Physical Activities and Sports for Healthy U.S. Adults by
Intensity of Effort

Light Activity (<3.0 METs or <4 kcal/min)	Moderate Activity (3.0–6.0 METs or 4–7 kcal/min)	Vigorous Activity (>6.0 METs or >7 kcal/min)
Archery	Basketball, non-game play	Basketball, game play
Billiards	Canoeing/kayaking/ rowing (2–3.9 mph)	**Boxing**
Bowling	Cycling (<10 mph)	Canoeing/kayaking/rowing (>4 mph)
Croquet	**Fishing, standing/ casting**	Cross-country skiing
Fishing, sitting	**Golf (pulling/carrying clubs)**	Cycling (>10 mph)
Golfing using a power cart	**Home care, general cleaning**	**Fencing**
Hatha yoga for 30 min[41]	**Hunting (bow or gun) small game**	**Fishing, in stream**
Home care, carpet sweeping	**Leisurely ice skating**	Football
Horseback riding, walking pace	**Mowing lawn, power mower**	**Judo**
Horseshoe pitching	**Sailing**	**Mountain climbing**
Mowing lawn, riding mower	**Sledding**	**Moving furniture**
Music playing	**Square dancing**	**Mowing lawn, hand mower**
Shuffleboard	Swimming, moderate effort	Racquet sports
Walking slowly (1–2 mph)	**T'ai Chi Chuan**[42]	**Rope jumping (>60 skips/min)**
	Table tennis	Running (>12 min/mile pace)
	Walking briskly (3–4 mph)	**Snowshoeing**
		Soccer
		Swimming, front crawl
		Walking briskly uphill with a load

Source: Modified from Refs. 4 and 5.

This chapter will review how one can benefit from participation in any of the following popular sports: football, basketball, baseball, softball, soccer, skiing, racquet sports (tennis, squash, and racquetball), golf, rowing, hockey, martial arts, and endurance sports (running, cycling, and swimming).

Football

Currently many hours of television programming are devoted to college and professional level games. Football is played throughout this country at all ages and skill levels. Playing touch football uses six to ten METs of energy (Table 7.2).[4] It is likely that pick-up games played by weekend warriors will result in benefits similar to those obtained while participating in tackle football. Actually, the benefit to risk ratio for the sport may be more favorable if tackling is avoided.

Each position in football requires a different skill set, but all players develop increased running speed, increased vertical jumping ability, and overall increased strength and flexibility. Football players need to be quick to avoid being tackled while carrying the ball or to catch their opponent with the ball. The running involved in the game of football involves sprinting interspersed with bursts of turning and pivoting to shake the defensive tackler or catch the offensive player with the ball. Speed testing has been shown to accurately predict draft status of running backs, wide receivers, and defensive backs.[8] Although this increased speed has been studied at the highest levels of football tournament play, the amateur athlete who enjoys continued participation in the fast-paced game of football will likely develop increased running speed.

In order to catch the ball before their opponent, a football player must be able to leap vertically in the air. In fact, the ability to play football has been directly correlated with the ability to jump high in the air.[9] The muscles used in this activity are the hip extensors (gluteal muscles), knee extensors (quadriceps), and ankle plantar flexors (gastrocnemius and soleus muscles). Strength and conditioning coaches design their programs to enhance the power of these muscles. The obvious way to increase the strength of these muscles is weight-lifting. The most effective warm-up protocol for the vertical jump is thought to be the warm-up with weights.[10] Since the game of football requires increased height of vertical leap, it is likely that one will benefit from this skill if that individual practices this sport.

Coaches often prize their players with excellent motor coordination. Due to the fast-paced nature of turnovers in football and the difficulty in catching a moving object while running at top speed, increased agility has become a pivotal skill in the game of football. One needs to only turn on ESPN to view the ever-increasing size of the football player. Not only are players of the third millennium bigger, but they are faster and stronger, too. The balance between strength and speed may be better termed agility. One may not attain the lightening reflexes of the National Football League's finest, but playing football regularly will increase agility.

Basketball

Dr. James Naismith, a Canadian physical education teacher, invented basketball in 1891 in Springfield, Massachusetts. Since that time, basketball has grown tremendously in popularity. Over 30 million Americans play recreational basketball each year.[11] Increased participation in basketball is of particular benefit for women, as they face a higher risk of osteoporosis as compared to men of the same age.[12]

Since basketball is primarily a running game, aerobic fitness is very important for performance. Players utilize seven to twelve METs of energy while playing, slightly more than the energy requirement for football (Table 7.2).[4] Most elite basketball players have excellent cardiovascular fitness because of the frequent jumping as well as running. However, the level of fitness and health benefits may depend on the position a person plays.[13] Guards and forwards will have less body fat and better aerobic fitness compared to the taller and heavier centers. Centers have better explosive power and can jump higher than their lighter counterparts.

Basketball develops gluteal, quadriceps, and calf muscles strength. Frequent overhead basketball shooting strengthens shoulder muscles (deltoids) as well as triceps and forearm muscles. This sport requires short bursts of speed. Players have well-developed fast twitch muscles to accomplish this task. Like football, regular basketball competition increases agility. Basketball has been shown to increase bone denisty in the bones of the spine (vertebra) as well as the bones of the feet (os calcaneus).[12] Unfortunately, basketball is the sport most frequently associated with ankle sprain.[14] The use of a lace-up ankle brace or taping the ankle prior to play may prevent injury.

BASEBALL AND SOFTBALL

Commonly referred to as America's favorite pastime, baseball still thrives in this age of video games. An estimated 19 million children are involved in youth baseball in the United States alone, and its popularity continues to grow worldwide.[15] Softball descended from baseball and was first played in 1887. Over 33 million Americans play in organized baseball and softball leagues.[16] Baseball and softball are generally sedentary sports with sporadic bursts of activity. Players must be ready to give 100 percent effort during a play without the benefit of a gradual warming up. Since there is no sustained aerobic activity, no MET level has been established for baseball. Swiftness, agility, and speed are paramount in this sport. Not surprisingly, good baseball players tend to have excellent hand-eye coordination. The muscles around their throwing arm tend to be stronger as well depending on the position they play.

The forces placed on the shoulder and elbow joints when throwing a baseball or softball are considerable.[17,18] Pitchers especially place extreme forces on their shoulder and elbow when pitching. Many of the motions in a baseball pitch are considered some of the fastest movements in all of sports.[17] The throwing shoulder develops differently during the adolescent period in baseball pichers.[17–19] Athletes who start learning overhand pitching when they are adults may place themselves at increased risk of shoulder and elbow injuries.

Parents, players, coaches, and referees should monitor pitch counts and avoid having an athlete with arm fatigue continue pitching during youth baseball games to prevent shoulder and elbow injuries.[20-22]

SOCCER

One only needs to witness the frenzied fans that attend the World Cup tournaments to appreciate the fact that soccer is arguably the most popular sport in the world. The sport known as "soccer" in the United States and "football" in other parts of the world dates back to as early as second and third centuries BC in China and possibly earlier.[23] Organized modern soccer began in England in 1863. In the United States alone, over 16 million Americans play soccer recreationally.[11] Unlike sports such as American football and basketball, teams may not call for time-outs and only the referee can call for temporary stoppages.[24]

Soccer requires excellent strength in the trunk and lower extremities.[24] The aerobic challenges of this sport combine the endurance requirements of a distance runner with the abrupt acceleration demands of a sprinter. Elite level mid-field male soccer players cover an average of 10 km (or 6.2 miles) during a game with sprinting comprising 10 percent of the distance covered. The number of METs expended playing soccer range from five METs (moderate activity) in a leisurely game to twelve METs (vigorous activity) in a more competitive environment (Table 7.2).[4] Soccer results in cardiovascular benefits and weight control. Also, athletes who play soccer regularly develop excellent agility and proprioceptive skills in order to make quick directional changes. However, pivoting during the game of soccer may cause injury to the ligaments of the knee. Although uncommon, collision injuries may occur during soccer. In fact, the American Academy of Pediatrics classifies soccer as a contact sport.[24]

SKIING

Skiing enjoys its greatest popularity in males under the age of thirty.[25] Since inertia reduces the amount of energy that comes from the skier, downhill skiing expends less METs than cross-country skiing (Table 7.2). Cross-country skiing expends four to greater than twelve METs.[4] Skiing on a flat surface is hard work that improves the ability of the body to utilize oxygen. This results in a superior cardiovascular benefit. In fact, cross-country skiers have an efficiency of oxygen utilization comparable to that of long distance runners. Of note, skiers have greater upper body strength than that of runners. Mean upper body power of runners is less than half of that of skiers.[26] Upper body strengthening is an important benefit of skiing that is often overlooked in standard exercise regimens. Like soccer, a common skiing injury is knee sprain or ligament tear. Consequently, proper knee extensor strengthening is important when beginning a ski program for exercise.

RACQUET SPORTS: TENNIS, SQUASH, AND RACQUETBALL

Tennis is a popular sport for all age participants. Over 22 million Americans play tennis recreationally.[27] Sports enthusiasts who can no longer tolerate the frequent collisions in football or jumping in basketball often turn to tennis for continued vigorous activity. The energy required to play tennis averages just below that of touch football (six to ten METs) and basketball (seven to twelve METs) at four to nine METs (Table 7.2).[4] To date, no research group has followed a group of tennis players throughout their lives as compared to a control group. However, studies have compared groups of tennis players of varying ages with age-matched sedentary controls. Senior tennis players demonstrate improved reaction time, greater bone density, greater strength, lower body fat, and enhanced aerobic capacity.[27]

The medical community has observed decreased reaction time with age as evidenced by increased falls in the elderly. Playing tennis may be one way to combat this problem.[28] Weight-bearing exercise improves bone health. Researches have evaluated this finding in tennis players. Initially, tennis players were found to have increased bone density in the bones of the dominant playing arm. This was thought to be related to increase muscle strength in the serving arm and has been demonstrated in both sexes. There is a similar phenomenon in the lumbar spine thought to be related to torsional stresses while playing tennis.[27] Tennis has been correlated with improved overall bone health as well. Critical analysis of the literature does suggest that male tennis players may benefit more than females in terms of overall improved bone density. Women have accelerated bone density loss after menopause. Weight-bearing exercise can help combat this problem.

Any aerobic exercise will lead to lower body fat and enhanced aerobic capacity. Tennis players who played twice a week for at least ten years achieved these benefits. These tennis players had lower body fat composition. Also, they may have more favorable lipid profiles. Although research has consistently demonstrated decreased body fat, studies of cholesterol values yielded variable results. This suggests genetic and other lifestyle factors may be at play. All exercise results in improved aerobic capacity. The average MET level for a game of tennis is seven (Table 7.2).[27] As previously mentioned, most sources regard greater than six METs as vigorous intense or high-impact physical activity. This type of activity burns seven kilocalories or more per minute.[25] Similar health benefits can be seen with playing racquetball and squash on a regular basis.

Playing tennis requires exceptional grip strength and the ability to resist the force of the ball on the racquet while keeping the wrist in neutral. Tennis players have better grip strength than nontennis players. As mentioned above, the influence from stronger muscles of the dominant arm is likely related to stronger bones. In addition to swinging a racquet, tennis requires strength of the muscles of the quadriceps and knee flexors (commonly called the hamstrings). There is debate about whether playing tennis results in stronger lower limb muscles. Tennis players do have increased strength of the lower limb muscles, but they also demonstrate increased knee injuries.[27] Another common injury in tennis is pain at the insertion of the wrist extensors at the elbow—termed "tennis elbow" or technically called lateral epicondylitis. This may be prevented with stretching of these muscles prior to play. Working on stroke technique may also be useful in someone prone to this injury.

GOLF

Invented in the twelfth century, golf is one of the most popular recreational activities in the United States. Approximately 20 million Americans play golf at least two times per year.[29] Although considered a sedentary sport, cardio-vascular benefits can be attained in golf. A recent study showed that golfers who walked the full eighteen holes of the course meet the recommendation to accumulate 10,000 steps per day as part of a general physical activity to improve a person's physical fitness.[30] In fact, during an eighteen-hole round, a golfer may walk more than 4 miles depending on the course lay-out. Another study showed that middle-aged male golfers who played golf two to three times per week and walked the golf course during their games lost upto one inch off their waist, had better cardiorespiratory fitness, and had an increase in HDL cholesterol over a five-month period of time.[31]

Walking a hilly golf course can exceed the recommendations for exercise placed by the ACSM.[32] A study on female golf caddies showed that they had better hand-grip and quadriceps strength as well as better bone density measurement in their heel.[33] One method for golfers who have difficulty walking the full course may be to alternate between walking a hole and using the cart for a hole or walking the first nine holes and using a cart for the final nine holes. The increased benefit of walking is reflected by the energy used. Utilization of a golf cart while playing requires only two to three METs (Table 7.2). Walking the course during the game will require four to seven METs.[2]

If done properly, swinging a golf club can build shoulder, forearm, upper back, pectoral, abdominal and "core" muscles, as well as gluteal, quadriceps and hamstring muscles. Carrying your bag while walking the course will increase the amount of cardiovascular work you will do. It may also place increased pressure on your back. If you have back problems, use golf bags with wheels or find other ways to transport your clubs to each hole without having to carry them while walking the course. Golfer's elbow, technically called medial epicondyltis, is somewhat similar to tennis elbow and may improve with gentle stretching and working on stroke technique.

ROWING

A slow Sunday paddle in a canoe and a champion crew team in major com-petition span the spectrum of this sport. Different muscles are used depending on the type of craft and the number of rowers involved. Of note, the speed of the boat does not increase proportionally with additional rowers. For example, a boat with two people does not go twice as fast as a boat with one rower. Thomas McMahon, a researcher at Harvard, discovered the factor by which speed increases per rower added to the boat.[34]

Since the buoyancy of water counterbalances the effect of weight, successful rowers typically weigh more than their peers. For example, rowing and cycling both require three to eight METs of energy (Table 7.2).[4] Greater body mass while cycling encourages greater air resistance. Water can support more mass than air. Unlike larger cyclers, larger rowers have a competitive advantage.[34] As such, weight lifting is an important training component of the sport of rowing. Rowers need not worry about the resistance effect of their increased size. These athletes benefit from increased bone density, strength, and aerobic fitness.

One might surmise that rowers show increased bone density in their dominant arm, similar to the finding in tennis players. However, the local effect is actually in their spine.[35] Strong bones occur in association with strong muscles. Rowing takes very strong lumbar paraspinal muscles. These muscles serve to extend the spine. In rowing, it is the muscles surrounding the spine in the low back that must do the most work. This finding accounts for increased bone density in the lumbar spine in rowers.

Rowers also have increase respiratory capacity related to their larger size.[34] Larger rowers experience little relative effect of increased wind and water resistance. As such, aerobic fitness is a better determinant of success in rowing. Thus, rowers benefit from increased cardiovascular efficiency. Regular rowing practice improves intake of oxygen and its extraction from the blood. The entire vascular system benefits from rowing. One study has shown increased fibrinolytic activity in rowers.[36] This demonstrated improved vascular efficiency. Rowing can improve the function of heart, lungs, and even blood vessels.

In addition to the muscles of the lumbar spine, rowing strengthens the muscles of the shoulder, hip, and knee. Powerful strokes start with increased power of the knee extensors and hip extensors. The hip flexors are involved because of their attachment on the lumbar spine and their relationship to pelvic tilt and the curve of the spine. Researchers have found that rowers exhibit increased lower limb strength overall as compared to other elite athletes.[37] The rotator cuff muscles of the shoulder as well as the arm and wrist flexors and extensors manipulate the paddles. Like cross-country skiers, people who enjoy rowing will benefit from increased strength of these upper extremity muscles. In fact, a modified rowing technique is often part of the physical therapy for strengthening of the rotator cuff after injury.

HOCKEY

Hockey players are adept at sustaining frequent physical contact while speed skating. The rapid changes in direction and velocity during a hockey game lead to increased lower extremity strength and improved endurance. Ice-skating builds strength of the lower extremity muscles. This can be observed in the enormous quadriceps and hamstrings of Olympic speed skaters. Elite hockey players show gains in endurance after one season of hockey play.[38] Unfortunately, collision injuries can sometimes occur during a hockey game. Numbness and tingling after collision injury, often called a "stinger" or a "burner," that does not resolve spontaneously should be evaluated by a physician.

MARTIAL ARTS

The term "martial arts" encompasses a spectrum from the slow movements of Tai Chi to the rapid punching and kicking of karate. Gripping and throwing techniques characterize Judo, the only martial art with an established MET level. This requires five to greater than ten METs. Soo bahk do utilizes both the slow and rapid techniques of the other styles. The benefits derived from martial arts depend upon the focus of the individual art. The purposeful movements of Tai Chi improve balance. Karate and tai kwon do practitioners develop increased muscle strength and flexibility. Participation in Soo bahk do elevates endurance levels and diminishes body fat. Nearly all styles result in cardiovascular benefit.[39]

ENDURANCE SPORTS

Running, cycling, and swimming are more frequently performed for exercise than any of the other organized sports mentioned in this chapter.[25] Much of what we know about the benefits of these activities comes from studying triathletes who are trying to enhance their performance. Success in a triathlon is directly correlated with the ability to sustain a high rate of energy throughout the competition.[40]

Of the three events, running requires the most energy at eight to sixteen METs (Table 7.2).[4] Unlike other sports, the MET level for running has been studied exhaustively due to the uniformity of activity. For example, running a six-minute mile requires 16.3 METs.[4] Swimming requires four to eight or more METs and cycling requires three to eight or more METs. This energy is in kilograms per minute and does not take distance into account. Of note, triathlons involve cycling a longer distance than running and running a longer distance than swimming because of different levels of fatigue associated with these activities. Similar to other sports, athletes who participate in triathlons demonstrate improved cardiovascular efficiency and lower body fat. Also, they develop the added benefit of increased upper body strength from swimming. As mentioned previously, upper body strengthening is often overlooked in standard fitness routines.

Runners and cyclists tend to be lean and may be tall. In contrast, swimmers are often very muscular. Tall runners and cyclists enjoy increased stride length. Shorter cyclists have the benefit of lower body mass, which may be particularly critical if their course involves hills. Due to their lean bodies, endurance athletes might not have the benefit of increased bone density seen in other sports. Runners are most at risk for stress fractures. Stress fractures occur when abnormal bone is exposed to repetitive stress, such as running long distances. Adding swimming to this equation may not improve bone density as swimming does not involve skeletal loading. Female runners or triathletes with foot or shin pain and decreased frequency of menses should be evaluated for stress fracture.

There is no doubt that sports convey tremendous health benefits to those who participate; however, these are dependent on many factors including the particular sport, intensity of play, and the athlete's physique. Of course, there are considerable injury risks for athletes—the most serious of which are usually seen in contact sports or those that involve high speed and acceleration.

REFERENCES

1. Paffenbarger Ralph S, Hyde RT, Wing AL, Lee IM, Jung DL, Kampert JB. "The Association of Changes in Physical-Activity Level and Other Lifestyle Characteristics with Mortality among Men." *New England Journal of Medicine* 328 (1993): 538–545.

2. Brill PA, Burkhalter HE, Kohl HW, Blair SN, Goodyear NN. "The Impact of Previous Athleticism on Exercise Habits, Physical Fitness, and Coronary Heart Disease Risk Factors in Middle-Aged Men." *Res Q Exerc Sport* 60 (1989): 209–215.

3. Pihl E, Jurimae T, Kaasik T. "Coronary Heart Disease Risk Factors in Middle-Aged Former Top Level Athletes." *Scan J Med Sci Sports* 8 (1998): 229–235.

4. Mahler Donald A et al. "General Principles of Exercise Prescription." In *American College of Sports Medicine Guidelines for Exercise Testing and Prescription*, edited by W Larry Kenney, Reed H Humphrey, and Cedric X Bryant (Philadelphia, PA: Williams and Wilkins, 1995), 153–176.

5. Pate Russell P et al. "Physical Activity and Public Health—A Recommendation from the Centers for Disease Control and Prevention and the American College of Sports Medicine." *Journal of the American Medical Association* 273 (1995): 402–407.

6. Kravitz Len, Vella C. "Energy Expenditure in Different Modes of Exercise." *American College of Sports Medicine Current Comment* (2002). http://www.acsm.org (accessed May 26, 2007).

7. American College of Sports Medicine Position Stand. "The Recommended Quantity of Exercise for Developing and Maintaining Cardiorespiratory and Muscular Fitness, and Flexibility in Healthy Adults." *Medicine and Science in Sports and Exercise* 30 (1998): 975–991.

8. McGee Kimberly J and Burkett Lee N. "The National Football League Combine: A Reliable Predictor of Draft Status." *The Journal of Strength and Conditioning Research* 17 (2003): 6–11.

9. Sawyer Donald T et al. "Relationship between Football Playing Ability and Selected Performance Measures." *The Journal of Strength and Conditioning Research* 16 (2002): 611–616.

10. Burkett Lee N, Phillips WT, Ziuraitis J. "The Best Warm-Up for the Vertical Jump in College-Age Athletic Men." *The Journal of Strength and Conditioning Research* 19 (2005): 673–676.

11. Cordell K et al. "Recreation Statistics Update: Trends in Activity Participation since Fall 1999." Southern Research Station and USDA Forest Service. http://www.srs.fs.fed.us/trends (accessed May 26, 2007).

12. Wolman RL. "ABC of Sports Medicine: Osteoporosis and Exercise." *British Medical Journal* 309 (1994): 400.

13. Ostojic SM, Mazic S, Dikic N. "Profiling in Basketball: Physical and Physiological Characteristics of Elite Players." *The Journal of Strength and Conditioning Research* 20 (2006): 740–744.

14. Conn JM, Annest JL, Gilchrist J. "Sports and Recreation Related Injury Episodes in the US Population, 1997–99." *Inj Prev* 9 (2003): 117–123.

15. Morales James R, Cardone Dennis A. "Baseball." In *Sports Medicine: Just the Facts*, edited by Francis G O'Connor, Robert E Sallis, Robert P Wilder, and Patrick St. Pierre (New York: McGraw-Hill, 2005), 461–464.

16. Flyger Nicholas, Button Chris, Rishiraj Neetu. "The Science of Softball: Implications for Performance and Injury Prevention." *Sports Medicine* 36 (2006): 797–816.

17. Fleisig Glenn S, Escamilla Rafael F, Barrentine Steven W. "Biomechanics of Pitching: Mechanism and Motion Analysis." In *Injuries in Baseball*, edited by James R Andrews, Bertram Zarins, and Kevin E Wilk (Philadelphia, PA: Lippincott-Raven Publishers, 1998), 3–22.

18. Crockett Heber C et al. "Osseous Adaptation and Range of Motion at the Glenohumeral Joint in Professional Baseball Pitchers." *The American Journal of Sports Medicine* 30 (2002): 20–26.

19. Osbahr Daryl C, Cannon David L, Speer Kevin P. "Retroversion of the Humerus in the Throwing Shoulder of College Baseball Pitchers." *The American Journal of Sports Medicine* 30 (2002): 347–353.

20. Meister Keith et al. "Rotational Motion Changes in the Glenohumeral Joint of the Adolescent/Little League Baseball Player." *The American Journal of Sports Medicine* 33 (2005): 693–698.

21. Lyman Samuel et al. "Effect of Pitch Type, Pitch Count and Pitching Mechaincs on Risk of Elbow and Shoulder Pain in Youth Baseball Pitchers." *The American Journal of Sports Medicine* 30 (2002): 463–468.

22. Olsen Samuel J II et al. "Risk Factors for Shoulder and Elbow Injuries in Adolescent Baseball Pitchers." *The American Journal of Sports Medicine* 34 (2006): 905–912.

23. Gerhardt Wilfred. "More Than 2000 Years of Football: The Colourful History of a Fascinating Game." Fédération Internationale de Football Association. http://www.fifa.com/fifa/history (accessed May 26, 2007).

24. Piantanida Nicholas A. "Soccer." In *Sports Medicine: Just the Facts*, edited by Francis G O'Connor, Robert E Sallis, Robert P Wilder, and Patrick St. Pierre. (New York: McGraw-Hill 2005), 526–531.

25. U.S. Department of Health and Human Services. *Physical Activity and Health: A Report of the Surgeon General*. Atlanta: U.S. Department of Health and Human Services, Centers for Disease Control and Prevention National Center for Chronic Disease Prevention and Health Promotion, 1996.

26. Gaskill SE, Serfass RC, Rundell KW. "Upper Body Power Comparison between Groups of Cross-Country Skiers and Runners." *International Journal of Sports Medicine* 20 (1999): 290–294.

27. Marks BL. "Health Benefits for Veteran Senior Tennis Players." *British Journal of Sports Medicine* 40 (2006): 469–476.

28. Rotella RJ, Bunker LK. "Field Dependence and Reaction Time in Senior Tennis Players." *Percept Mot Skills.* 46 (1978): 585–586.

29. Dammann Gregory G, Levy Jeffrey A. "Golfing Injuries." In *Sports Medicine: Just the Facts,* edited by Francis G O'Connor, Robert E Sallis, Robert P Wilder, and Patrick St. Pierre (New York: McGraw-Hill, 2005), 497–500.

30. Kobriger Samantha L et al. "The Contribution of Golf to Daily Physical Activity Recommendations: How Many Steps Does It Take to Complete a Round of Golf." *Mayo Clinic Proceedings* 81 (2006): 1041–1043.

31. Parkkari Jari et al. "A Controlled Trial of the Health Benefits of Regular Walking on a Golf Course." *The American Journal of Medicine* 109 (2000):102–108.

32. Stauch M, Liu Y, Giesler M, Lehmann M. "Physical Activity Level during a Round of Golf on a Hilly Course." *Journal of Sports Medicine and Physical Fitness* 39 (1999): 321–317.

33. Hoshino H et al. "Effect of Physical Activity as a Caddie on Ultrasound Measurements of the Os Calcis: A Cross-Sectional Comparison." *Journal of Bone and Mineral Research* 11 (1996): 412–418.

34. Zumerchik J. *Encyclopedia of Sports Science* (New York: Simon and Schuster Macmillan, 1997), 333–334.

35. Wolman RL, Clark P, McNally E, Harries M, Reeve J. "Menstrual State and Exercise as Determinants of Spinal Trabecular Bone Density in Female Athletes." *British Medical Journal* 301 (1990): 516–518.

36. Cerneca E, Simeone R, Bruno G, Gombacci A. "Coagulation Parameters in Senior Athletes Practicing Endurance Sporting Activity." *Journal of Sports Medicine and Physical Fitness* 45 (2005): 576–579.

37. Hagerman FC. "Applied Physiology of Rowing." *Sports Med* 4 (1984): 303–326.

38. Montgomery DL. "Physiology of Ice Hockey." *Sports Med* 5 (1988): 99–126.

39. Douris P, Chinan A, Gomez M, Aw A, Steffens D, Weiss S. "Fitness Levels of Middle Aged Martial Art Practitioners." *British Journal of Sports Medicine* 38 (2004): 143–147.

40. O'Toole ML, Douglas PS. "Applied Physiology of Triathlon." *Sports Med* 19 (1995): 251–267.

41. Clay Carolyn et al. "The Metabolic Cost of Hatha Yoga." *The Journal of Strength and Conditioning Research* 19 (2005): 604–610.

42. Schneider D and Leung R. "Metabolic and Cardiorespiratory Responses to the Performance of Wing Chun and T'ai Chi Chuan Exercises." *International Journal of Sports Medicine* 12 (1991): 319–323.

8

Exercise and Obesity

Daniel S. Rooks and George L. Blackburn

History

We are in the midst of an international obesity epidemic brought on by several decades of overeating and declining physical activity. Over the past twenty years, obesity has grown so prevalent it has surpassed undernutrition and infectious disease and may soon overtake smoking as the major risk factor for chronic illness, morbidity, and premature mortality.[1] In 2005, approximately 400 million adults worldwide were obese and 1.6 billion were overweight. The number of obese is predicted to increase by 75 percent (700 million) by the year 2015.[2] In the United States, the number of obese has quadrupled since 1990. Currently, two thirds of Americans are obese (32.2%) or overweight (34.1%). The most severely obese, those individuals having more than 100 pounds of excess body weight are the fastest growing portion of the obese population having increased in number fivefold in the past fifteen years. Mirroring this rapid rise in adults has been a doubling and tripling of the number of obese children and adolescents, respectively.[3] A graphical presentation of the growth of obesity in the United States can be seen at the Center for Disease Control and Prevention Web site.[3]

Defined as an unhealthy excess of body fat, obesity is a chronic disease that can have a severely negative effect on health. The additional fat can dramatically increase the chance of suffering from a chronic illness of one or more body systems and can seriously compromise emotional health, well-being, and quality of life. Obese individuals commonly experience chronic illness at an earlier age compared with normal and even overweight adults. Obesity is a major risk factor for cardiovascular diseases such as heart disease, high blood pressure and stroke, arthritis and other musculoskeletal disorders, several cancers, type 2 diabetes, and sleep apnea. Not surprising, the number of American children with chronic health problems, including obesity and obesity-related issues, has quadrupled in the past thirty to forty years.[4] This increase in the prevalence of childhood chronic illness is the cause of great concern because it predicts a similar rise in severe illness and premature disability in young adulthood; all of this occurring at a much earlier age than what has previously been seen. The problem of obesity has spawned a subsequent epidemic of diabetes, together, which threaten to reverse for the first time in centuries, the life expectancy of current generations.

Chronic illness is costly from both a financial and human perspective causing significant health and nonhealth related expenses and disability. Approximately three quarters of the United States' trillion dollar health-care expenses are related to chronic illness.[5,6] Health-related costs of obesity, which include greater use of medication and health care resources, are reported to be more than $139 billion annually and growing.[7] Obesity is estimated to cause at least 300,000 deaths a year.

While genetics plays a role, the exponential rise in the prevalence of obesity in the past three decades is due in large part to an increase in the availability and consumption of nutritionally poor, calorie-dense foods and a decrease in physical activity. In addition to the higher calorie content of foods, there has been a "portion distortion"[8,9] where a single serving size has increased dramatically, for example soda has risen from 10 oz to 16–24 oz and bagels from 3.5″ to 5–6″ in diameter. Today, the average diet contains fewer fruits, vegetables, and whole grains and more sugar and fat. People are also eating out more often, particularly at fast food restaurants. Several years ago, it was reported that the average American eats 140 pounds more food per year than a decade ago. This includes approximately 25 pounds of sugar per person.[10]

Concurrent with dietary changes, industrialized societies have successfully engineered physical activity out of many aspects of daily life. Labor-saving devices at work and at home, more sedentary job tasks (i.e., word processing, e-mail), and the evolution of the home for entertainment and recreation (i.e., television, video game systems, growth of cable networks) has reallocated our time to more sedentary activities. Today, you don't even have to turn on a faucet, push the soap dispenser, or manually dry your hands if you don't want to. You can step onto a "moving walkway" in many airports and use escalators instead of taking the stairs. All of these, while convenient, systematically remove small amounts of physical activity from the day and contribute to a less physically active lifestyle. The challenge in the current "obesogenic" environment is that an average daily net increase of only 100 calories can lead to an annual 10-pound weight gain. Therefore, elimination of any daily energy expenditure puts a person at risk for weight gain. Independent of weight gain, physical inactivity is thought to cause approximately one quarter of ischemic heart disease and 10 to 16 percent of certain types of cancer (breast, colon, rectum) and type 2 diabetes.[11] Consequently, we must consciously add physical activity into our day to help counterbalance this shift toward a net gain in calories.

The "set point" theory defines the challenge of weight management; the body adapts to maintain a certain body weight. Evolutionarily, the brain becomes programmed or "set" at a particular weight. This usually occurs when you remain at a certain weight for an extended period. When food is plentiful, the body stores calories above those needed for daily activity as body fat. Alternatively, when food is scarce the body reduces the amount of calories it needs to maintain normal function. The body's sensitive adjustment to the environment allows for the cyclical periods of starvation and plentiful food seen during the "hunting and gathering" period of evolution and probably developed to improve survival. Metabolism is the amount of energy used by the body to maintain its many functions. With a low food intake, the body believes it is in a period of starvation and lowers the metabolism to spare muscle and other tissues.

Remembering that our genome is still programmed to defend a certain body weight or "set point," fast forward to today where two common scenarios occur. The first is that most people do not have to contend with the cycle of starvation and plenty, often consuming more calories than are needed to maintain their body weight. Concurrent with this is a decline in the amount of physical activity that helps maintain the energy balance. The resulting gradual weight gain continuously "resets" the weight point the body thinks is needed for survival and encourages the body to eat to sustain that ever-increasing body weight. The second scenario deals with the yo-yo pattern of dieting where people fluctuate between severely reducing the amount of calories they consume daily for several weeks, then returning to their normal diet. Does this second scenario sound familiar? It resembles the starvation–plenty cycle of our ancestors that activates the survival mechanism causing the body to protect the set point body weight. This is one reason why trying to lose large amounts of weight quickly is difficult and typically not sustained. The lesson learned is to work with the body's systems, not against them to successfully lose body fat; achieve a healthy body weight with a new set point and become more physically fit. Habitual exercise and physical activity are critical to these aspects of successful weight management. This chapter describes the role of exercise in a weight management program.

DIAGNOSIS

Obesity is often characterized by the location of fat deposits on the body. General obesity is seen with fat deposited throughout the body and is often described as the "pear shape" appearance where deposits of fat are centralized in the hips, thighs, and buttocks areas. Abdominal obesity, described as the "apple shape," refers to a fat distribution centralized on the abdomen. Abdominal obesity has been shown to represent the deposit of fat under the skin (subcutaneous) and within and among the organs of the abdomen (intra-abdominal) and is associated with greater health risks.

The most commonly used indicator of obesity for large populations is *body mass index* (BMI), which assesses weight for height. BMI is defined as the body weight in kilograms divided by the height in meters squared (weight in kg/height in m^2). If you prefer to use pounds and inches instead of kilograms and meters, divide body weight in pounds by the person's height in inches squared and multiply the answer by 703 (lbs./in^2 × 703). BMI can be calculated quickly and easily at several public health Web sites, for example www.nhlbisupport.com/bmi, http://www.cdc.gov/nccdphp/dnpa/bmi/index.htm. BMI is used internationally as a screening tool and a general indicator of body fatness. The World Health Organization (WHO) classifies a person with a BMI of >30 as obese.[1]

While BMI is the most widely accepted measure for obesity, the threshold of 30 may not be universally accurate. It has been suggested that people of Asian decent may be obese at a BMI of closer to 25. Furthermore, at the same BMI, the percentage of body fat may differ based on sex, age, and fitness level. Women may have a higher percentage of body fat than men at the same BMI due to normal gender-based fat distribution differences. Older adults typically loose muscle mass as they age. Therefore, at the same BMI, older adults may have higher levels of body fat than younger adults. Finally, very physically fit individuals, such as competitive athletes, typically have higher levels of muscle mass and lower percentages of body fat than nonathletes, yet by BMI, they are classified as overweight (BMI = 25 to 29.9). The term *overweight* refers to a body weight above that of national standards and is not specifically associated with body fat. Classifying obesity and overweight in children and adolescents is less clear because of the lack of a universally accepted definition, which is an area of current research.

Independent of total body fat, an excess amount of fat in and around the abdomen is an additional health risk in people with a BMI between 25 and 34.9 kg/m^2. This increased danger is associated with a greater chance of developing type 2 diabetes, cardiovascular disease, high cholesterol, and high blood pressure and their related consequences.[12-14] The most practical approach to assessing the presence of abdominal fat is to use waist circumference, measured above the hips at the level of the waist. Holding a tape measure around the back just above the pelvic bones and level to the floor, both ends are moved to the front of the abdomen and recorded in inches or centimeters. The highest health risk is in men with a waist circumference above 40 inches and in women above 35 inches (Table 8.1).[15,16]

Body composition, the amount and percent of muscle, bone, and fat on the body, can be measured more precisely using technology. These measures are not commonly used due to cost or limited accessibility. Dual-energy x-ray absorptiometry (DEXA) used to measure bone density can calculate the amount of body fat. Bioelectrical impedance is a method of determining body fat by measuring the difference in the rate at which an electric current goes from one point on the body to another. The impedance of the electrical signal for fat and muscle differ, thereby allowing the determination of the percentage of each type of tissue in the body. Skinfold thickness, a less precise method of estimating body fatness requires the direct measurement of the thickness of skin or fat folds at specific locations on the body, a trained person to take the measurements and the use of scientifically developed formulae.

Table 8.1
Body Mass Index (BMI) Classifications, Waist Circumference, and Associated
Disease Risk*

	BMI (kg/m^2)	Disease Risk Associated with Waist Circumference: Men ≤102 cm (≤40 in.) Women ≤88 cm (≤35 in.)	Disease Risk Associated with Waist Circumference: Men >102 cm (>40 in.) Women >88 cm (>35 in.)
Underweight	18.5	—	—
Normal+	18.5–24.9	—	—
Overweight	25.0–29.9	Increased	High
Obesity	30.0–34.9	High	Very High
	35.0–39.9	Very High	Very High
Extreme or Severe Obesity	≥40	Extremely High	Extremely High

*Increased risk for type 2 diabetes, hypertension, and CVD.
+Larger waist circumference can also be a marker for increased risk even in persons of normal weight.
Source: Modified from Obesity Education Initiative of the National Institutes of Health (NIH) at http://www.nhlbi.nih.gov/guidelines/obesity/e_txtbk/txgd/4142.htm.

COMMON TREATMENT APPROACHES

Obesity is a complex health problem with physical, emotional, social, cultural, and other causes. In its simplest form, obesity is the result of an energy imbalance—more calories are consumed than are expended. Losing body fat requires a flip in the energy imbalance, where more calories are expended than are consumed. There are three primary approaches to losing body fat: eat less (reduce caloric consumption), be more physically active (increase caloric expenditure), or combine the two. The most popular approach to weight loss and management is restricting calorie consumption, also known as "dieting." Restricting calories below the level of energy needed during a day prompts the body to use body fat and other energy stores to provide the needed energy. The weight loss industry is a multibillion-dollar business providing a myriad of ways of reducing calories and using up body fat. The bookstore shelves are filled with a variety of diet programs named after the people who developed them, a principle food in the diet, the geographical area where it was developed, and others. Unfortunately, losing weight is very difficult for most people, with more than 95 percent of people who set out to lose weight not succeeding. Specifics about dietary modification are beyond the scope of this chapter. In general, the type of diet—low carbohydrate, low fat, predetermined balance of carbohydrates, proteins and fats, or exchange list diet—all can be effective for losing weight.[17] The critical factor is selecting a diet plan that meets your health needs and that you can stick with. To help determine what dietary approach may be best and to account for individual nutrition or health issues, discuss your interest in weight management with your physician or a dietician.

Hypothetically, exercise alone should lead to weight loss. However, the reality can be quite different. Let us say you exercise for one hour a day burning 350 calories during that time. If your food choices and portions are reasonable and remain the same, you would lose approximately one pound of fat every ten days (3,500 calories = 1 pound of fat). It is not easy or even feasible to assume that calorie intake will remain constant. On top of this, it is common for people who are trying to lose weight to think that exercising is permission for a larger portion or special dietary treat. With today's portions, it would not take much to eat an additional 350 calories. Therefore, combining physical activity and exercise with smart, healthy eating can allow for a safe 500-calorie deficit each day that can lead to a one-pound fat loss approximately every seven days. Additionally, combining healthy eating with exercise is the best way to improve short and long-term health and adopt a healthful lifestyle. It only takes a 10 percent weight loss to see important health benefits.

A habitual high level of physical activity is a recurring theme among many long-term studies that identify predictors of successful weight management. Several studies have reported that people who performed between 250 and 300 minutes of physical activity per week were the most successful at maintaining their weight loss long-term.[18,19] These data have led to the recommendations from the American College of Sports Medicine[20,21] and the 2005 U.S. Dietary Guidelines for Americans.[22,23]

To understand clearly the guidelines around exercise requires the definition of four terms. *Physical activity* is any bodily movement produced by skeletal muscles that results in an expenditure of energy.[24] *Exercise* is a subcategory of physical activity that is planned or structured and involves repetitive bodily movement done to improve or maintain one or more of the components of physical fitness—cardiorespiratory endurance (aerobic fitness), muscular strength, muscular endurance, flexibility, and body composition.[24] The amount of energy expended is dependent upon the intensity of effort and duration of the activity. Two terms differentiate the levels of intensity. *Moderate intensity physical activity* describes sustained rhythmic movements with the level of effort similar to walking briskly, dancing, or bicycling on level terrain. Typically, a person should feel some exertion but should be able to carry on a conversation comfortably during the activity. *Vigorous intensity physical activity* generally describes movements such as jogging, mowing the lawn with a push mower, swimming continuous laps, or bicycling up hill. This level of effort usually results in raising a person's heart and breathing rates.[24]

PRECAUTIONS

Obesity is associated with several chronic health conditions, such as diabetes and cardiovascular disease, which can be exacerbated by inappropriate exercise. Therefore, it is imperative that a person visit with his or her primary care doctor and other health professionals before starting any exercise program. A conversation about exercise should include what forms of exercise are appropriate and which are not safe for the individual. It is recommended that regular contact with the health care provider, whether in person or by other means (i.e., telephone or e-mail) occur for the initial twelve weeks of a program.

Most individuals with type 2 diabetes are obese and have additional precautions to address due to the disease process of diabetes and its associated comorbidities. Coronary artery disease, common in people with diabetes, must be assessed in individuals planning a program of moderately intense or vigorous exercise. Determination of whether to undergo a treadmill or bicycle stress test is the decision of the primary care physician and specialist. Additionally, exercise and physical activity can have an insulin-like action on blood sugar, which can cause low blood sugar (hypoglycemia) with too much insulin or high blood sugar (hyperglycemia) from too little. Therefore, individuals taking medication to regulate their blood sugar, particularly insulin injections, will likely have to regulate the amount and timing of their medication before and after exercise. Proper foot care and footwear are essential for the person with diabetes to exercise successfully. This aspect of diabetes self-management should be discussed with the health care provider or diabetes educator.

Associated with obesity, depression should be treated separately from weight management. The presence of depression, with or without obesity, can reduce a person's adherence to an exercise program. The combination of exercise, particularly in a group format, can be effective at improving mood and exercise participation.[25]

Other considerations include weather, particularly temperature. Fat is a very effective insulator. On hot days, an obese person may not be able to regulate body temperature adequately. It is best to exercise indoors during hotter weather where the air quality may also be better. The exercise program can be shortened or performed at a lower intensity on hot days. If one must be outside, it is best to be active during the cooler times of the day.

BARRIERS TO EXERCISE

The numerous barriers to exercise for the obese individual must be considered when designing an exercise program. Embarrassment is the primary reason obese or overweight people are hesitant to exercise. Many people are not comfortable participating in activities that require revealing clothing, such as a swimsuit, or bouncing. People may not have much experience performing physical activities that require skills and technique and are uncomfortable to ask for help. Additionally, many do not want to be part of programs or classes where other participants are very fit, are held in public places where people can stare, or that require changing in open locker rooms. For the severely obese, issues such as adequate sized benches and doorways, reinforced toilets, and sufficiently spacious shower stalls and changing areas are essential. Particular exercise movements may be uncomfortable or limited by body mass. People who have been large their entire life may not have many positive experiences with sports or exercise, such as being picked last for a team. Another obstacle is safety and the concern of having a heart attack or other medical emergency because of exercise. To address the issues a person must be comfortable with the activities of an exercise program, have a reliable source for learning the techniques of the activity, be comfortable with the location and environment where activities will be performed, and have knowledge that the instructor is able to adapt the activity to the limitations of a person of size.

Another common barrier to exercise is the inappropriate or poorly defined exercise program. This is seen when the person lacks specific guidance on what level of effort to exercise at and how often or how long each session should last. This is particularly relevant for the individual with little exercise experience. When less active people exercise too much, they typically experience excessive soreness in muscles and joints. This discomfort is referred to as *delayed onset muscle soreness* and is a common reason a person gives up exercising. If the exercise plan is not modified, the same thing will happen when the person starts to exercise again. The most common obstacle for exercising is not enough time. Therefore, any exercise plan must fit into a person's lifestyle and must be convenient. The goal of an exercise program for the obese individual is to initiate and sustain a lifestyle of habitual physical activity and exercise. This requires consideration of obstacles that prevent or deter regular exercise participation.

HEALTH BENEFITS OF EXERCISE

For the obese individual, habitual physical activity and exercise participation can benefit many aspects of life. The physical aspects of exercise are the most frequently stated and include immediate and long-term benefits. The body responds to a bout of exercise by increasing the metabolic rate, burning calories during and for up to twenty-four to forty-eight hours after exercise and increasing the blood supply to the heart, brain, muscles, bones, and other body systems. In response to exercising, the body starts to make changes to improve its use of oxygen, insulin, and other body substances including fats and cholesterol and to increase muscle strength and endurance. Therefore, if a person exercises on most days of the week, these *immediate* changes are *extended* for as long as exercise is performed regularly. These changes make up the small steps needed to bring about long-term improvements in fitness, health, and function. These physical changes can improve the symptoms and management of chronic illness, such as in diabetes and arthritis, delay or prevent the onset of certain diseases or injuries (i.e., diabetes, falls), and preserve functional capacity and independence.

Exercise can have a very powerful effect on a person's emotional health and well-being. As mentioned earlier, it is well accepted that habitual exercise can improve depression and other mental health conditions that are common with obesity. When performed in a class format, exercise can be a very social activity addressing the issue of isolation and loneliness often seen in obese individuals. As mentioned earlier, one barrier to exercise is being unfamiliar with how to perform exercises correctly and safely. After developing the skills and abilities to exercise independently, most people perceive greater progress and develop more motivation to keep exercising. Additionally, people who exercise regularly often feel emotional support for their accomplishments from other exercisers, friends, family, health care providers, and other members of their support network.

Participation in regular exercise can also bring about social and environmental benefits. Enjoyable exercise has a greater chance of being continued. For many individuals who experience society's contempt and isolation of the obese, exercise can be an important connection with a supportive social circle. Individuals who have used a particular type of exercise (i.e., water aerobics, floor aerobics, strength training) to successfully manage their weight may become trained to lead exercise classes and help others with the goal of weight loss. Environmental health benefits include reducing air and noise pollution and automotive traffic congestion when choosing to walk or use other forms of physical activity as transportation.

EXERCISE PRESCRIPTION

The goal of any exercise program for weight management is to reduce body fat stores, preserve muscle mass, and improve overall health and body function. For long-term success, the program must increase energy expenditure, be enjoyable, convenient, and flexible to fit into a person's lifestyle. One of the most difficult challenges of becoming more physically active and starting an exercise program is knowing what to do and how often to do it. The remaining sections of this chapter will discuss these central issues.

In 2005, the latest guidelines for exercise for the purpose of weight management were released as part of the U.S. Dietary Guidelines for Americans.[23] These are the first dietary guidelines to include language that encourages regular physical activity and the reduction of sedentary behavior to promote health, psychological well-being, and a healthy body weight. The guidelines address three levels of health. The first, to reduce the risk of chronic disease, suggests at least thirty minutes of moderate intensity physical activity at work or at home on most days of the week. The second, to help manage body weight and prevent gradual body weight gain, suggests approximately sixty minutes of moderate to vigorous physical activity at work or home on most days of the week. Finally, for sustaining weight loss in adulthood, daily physical activity of moderate to vigorous intensity for sixty to ninety minutes is recommended. These recommendations are based on research findings from large populations that include individuals who were obese, had pre-diabetes or impaired glucose tolerance (decreased ability to process sugar from the blood to the muscles), and who lost 70 pounds or more and kept it off for longer than three years.[26,27]

For most individuals who are obese, becoming more physically active is an important first step toward starting and enjoying a regular exercise program. With a little creativity, physical activity can be added to anybody's daily life. Parking farther from work or a store and walking the additional distance is the most common suggestion. For the person who has trouble walking, the grocery store can be a safe place to begin. Holding on to a cart for support, you can walk all or some of the aisles. Carry one or two bags at a time when bringing grocery bags into the home. Instead of taking the elevator all the way to your floor, walk one flight of stairs and take the elevator the rest of the way. After two to three weeks of this, walk two flights and ride the rest of the way. Continue this pattern and in time, you may be able to walk all the stairs. Do not use automatic door openers unless you need to; the calories used to push or pull doors open add up. House and yard work are good ways to burn calories. Next to walking, gardening is the most popular form of physical activity in the United States and a wonderful hobby. Walk to a nearby store instead of drive, or go visit a neighbor instead of calling on the telephone.

An exercise program should be planned to meet a person's individual likes and dislikes, needs and goals for maximum safety and effectiveness. When developing a program, each exercise should follow the FITT-P guideline. *Frequency* refers to how often to exercise. *Intensity* is the level of effort exerted to perform the exercise. Moderate intensity is sufficient to successfully manage weight, maintain muscle mass, and gain the many health benefits from exercise. *Type* refers to what exercise you perform, that is walking, cycling, dancing, swimming. *Time* is how much time you spend on aerobic exercises and how many repetitions of strength training activities you perform. *Progression* is how to increase safely the amount of exercise performed to improve fitness.

Before starting any exercise program, be sure to check with your primary care physician, as well as any other health professional you see regularly to make sure the program is appropriate for you and identify activities you should avoid. The right amount of exercise will make a person feel good and provide the best chance to achieve the goal of losing body fat and maintaining a healthy weight. Too much exercise can make your muscles very sore and tired and increase the risk of injury. Too little exercise can lead to a loss of interest due to a lack of improvement.

AEROBIC EXERCISE

Walking is an important part of everyday life and a preferred form of physical activity and exercise. It is recommended that aerobic exercise be performed three to five times per week.[20] Monitoring and attending the intensity of aerobic exercise can be done simply without high technology. A general rule is that you should walk (or perform any other aerobic activity) with a sense of determined purpose.[28,29] A way to monitor the effort during aerobic exercise is the *talk test*. This simple test says that if you are not able to carry on a conversation while exercising, you are pushing yourself too hard and should slow down. A more sophisticated method of assessing intensity is by monitoring heart rate. A training heart rate, the heart rate range used during exercise, is calculated using a simple formula (220 − age). An example of calculating training heart rate for a 45-year-old sedentary man or woman:

$$(220 - 45) \times .5 = 175 \times .5 = 88 \text{ beats per minute}$$
$$(220 - 45) \times .6 = 175 \times .6 = 105 \text{ beats per minute}$$

This 45-year-old should have a heart rate between 88 and 105 beats per minute while exercising.

Choosing your exercise is a matter of personal preference. Select something you enjoy doing; it increases your chance of staying with the exercise. The starting time is also an individual choice. Many heavy people cannot exercise for more than five to ten minutes without needing to stop and rest. In this case, the person should begin exercising for as long as he or she is comfortable, but stop before getting too fatigued. For example, a person may begin by walking for four minutes. During subsequent weeks, add thirty seconds to each walking session that week (four minutes thirty seconds in Week 2 and five minutes in Week 3). Continue adding thirty seconds each week until walking for ten minutes continuously. At ten minutes, one to two minutes per week can be added until the person is walking for thirty minutes continuously. The continuous progression of thirty seconds to one minute allows the body to adapt gently to the increase in exercise time.

STRENGTH TRAINING

Strength training exercise should be performed two to three times per week with at least forty-eight hours of rest between workouts. Aerobic exercise can be done on the same day or different days of the week as strength training exercise. Intensity for strength training exercise is determined by how much effort is required to perform the exercise movement. Strength training exercise is measured by the number of times an exercise is performed without resting. Performing an exercise one time is referred to as a *repetition* and a series of repetitions performed in sequence without resting is referred to as a *set*. Begin with one set of six to eight repetitions adding one or two repetitions each week until performing eight to twelve repetitions of an exercise. One set of eight to twelve repetitions at a moderate intensity is sufficient to increase muscle tone and strength. Exercises that involve the major muscles of the body should be included in an exercise program. Start with one or two exercises and add one exercise every two to three weeks, as you feel comfortable. A program of six to eight exercises works well.

FLEXIBILITY

Flexibility exercises can be performed daily and should be done at least four to five days each week. The purpose of these exercises is to increase the comfort range of movement of major joints—neck, shoulders, back, hips, knees, and ankles. Flexibility exercises, also referred to as *stretching*, should be done in a relaxed and gentle manner. Exercise selection and instruction can be found with a group class, DVD, or well-designed book. A choice of exercises can be made with the assistance of a physical therapist, qualified fitness professional, nurse, or physician. Hold movements for fifteen to thirty seconds and repeated twice. Group activities including Tai Chi and certain styles of yoga can be good alternatives.

Exercise is a critical component of a weight management plan. In addition to being a key source of energy expenditure, habitual exercise has a myriad of general health benefits for the obese individual, independent of age, sex, or the presence of comorbidities. A written program tailored to the individual's needs and preferences, identification of individual goals, and the presence of a social support network of family, friends and others gives a person the greatest chance of adopting a more active lifestyle that will facilitate successful weight management.

FUTURE CONSIDERATIONS

Obesity is a complex health crisis that requires a multipronged approach to prevention, treatment, and long-term weight loss maintenance on several levels. As a public health problem, we must address the issues through government policy, health care, the workplace, schools, community design, and promoting and empowering individual responsibilities. We live in a culture of "consumer convenience" with easily accessible and relatively inexpensive food and declining physical activity. Physical activity has been part of our genetic make-up from the beginning and an important component of general good health and well-being. We must consciously include physical activity and exercise in our daily lives to promote health, reduce the risk of chronic illness, and help derail the onrushing train that is the obesity epidemic.

REFERENCES

1. World Health Organization (2007a). *Obesity.* Retrieved June 28, 2007, from http://www.who.int/topics/obesity/en/.

2. World Health Organization (2007b). *Obesity Fact Sheet.* Retrieved July 11, 2007, from http://www.who.int/mediacentre/factsheets/fs311/en/index.html.

3. Center for Disease Control and Prevention (2007a). *Obesity.* Retrieved June 28, 2007, from http://www.cdc.gov/nccdphp/dnpa/obesity/.

4. Perrin JM, Bloom SR, Gortmaker SL. The increase of childhood chronic conditions in the United States. *JAMA* 297 (2007):2755–2759.

5. Catlin A, Cowan C, Heffler S, Washington B. National health spending in 2005: The slowdown continues. *Health Aff* 26 (2007):142–153.

6. Trends in aging—United States and worldwide. *MMWR* 52 (2003):101–104, 106.

7. Andersen LH, Martinson BC, Crain AL, et al. (October 2005). *Health Care Charges Associated with Physical Inactivity, Overweight, and Obesity,* from http://www.cdc.gov/pcd/issues/2005/oct/04_0118.htm.

8. National Heart Lung and Blood Institute, NIH, U.S. Department of Health and Human Services. *Portion Distortion.* Retrieved July 11, 2007, from http://hp2010.nhlbihin.net/portion/

9. Obesity in America: Large portions, large proportions. *Harvard Men's Health Watch* (2006).

10. Why do we eat so much? *Harvard Men's Health Watch* (November 2004).

11. World Health Organization (2007c). *Physical Activity.* Retrieved July 9, 2007, from http://www.who.int/topics/physical_activity/en/

12. Hu FB, Manson JE, Stampfer MJ, et al. Diet, lifestyle, and the risk of type 2 diabetes mellitus in women. *N Engl J Med* 345 (2001):790–797.

13. Katzmarzyk PT, Janssen I, Ardern CI. Physical inactivity, excess adiposity and premature mortality. *Obes Rev* 4 ((2003):257–290.

14. Tanaka K, Nakanishi T. Obesity as a risk factor for various diseases: Necessity of lifestyle changes for healthy aging. *Appl Human Sci* 15 (1996):139–148.

15. NHLBI Obesity Education Initiative Expert Panel. (1998). *Clinical Guidelines on the Identification, Evaluation, and Treatment of Overweight and Obesity in Adults: The Evidence Report.* Bethesda, MD: National Heart, Lung, and Blood Institute, NIH, U.S. Department of Health and Human Services.

16. *The Practical Guide: Identification, Evaluation, and Treatment of Overweight and Obesity in Adults* (No. NIH Publication 02-4084)(2000). Bethesda, MD: NHLBI and NAASO.

17. Dansinger ML, Gleason JA, Griffith JL, et al. Comparison of the Atkins, Ornish, Weight Watchers, and Zone diets for weight loss and heart disease risk reduction: a randomized trial. *JAMA* 293 (2005):43–53.

18. Jakicic JM, Clark K, Coleman E, et al. American College of Sports Medicine position stand. Appropriate intervention strategies for weight loss and prevention of weight regain for adults. *Med Sci Sports Exerc* 33 (2001):2145–2156.

19. Sarlio-Lahteenkorva S, Rissanen A. Weight loss maintenance: Determinants of long-term success. *Eat Weight Disord* 3 (1998):131–135.

20. Haskell WL, Lee IM, Pate RR, et al. Physical activity and public health: Updated recommendation for adults from the American College of Sports Medicine and the American Heart Association. *Circulation* 116 (2007):1081–1093.

21. Nelson ME, Rejeski WJ, Blair SN, et al. Physical activity and public health in older adults: Recommendation from the American College of Sports Medicine and the American Heart Association. *Med Sci Sports Exerc* 39 (2007):1435–1445.

22. Blackburn GL, Waltman BA. Physician's guide to the new 2005 dietary guidelines: How best to counsel patients. *Cleve Clin J Med* 72 (2005):609–618.

23. U.S. Department of Health and Human Services, U.S. Department of Agriculture (2005). *Dietary guidelines for Americans 2005,* from http://www.healthierus.gov/dietaryguidelines/.

24. Center for Disease Control and Prevention (2007b). *Physical Activity Terms.* Retrieved May 26, 2007, from http://www.cdc.gov/nccdphp/dnpa/physical/terms/index.htm.

25. Penninx BW, Rejeski WJ, Pandya J, et al. Exercise and depressive symptoms: A comparison of aerobic and resistance exercise effects on emotional and physical function in older persons with high and low depressive symptomatology. *J Gerontol B Psychol Sci Soc Sci* 57 (2002):124–132.

26. Haffner S, Temprosa M, Crandall J, et al. Intensive lifestyle intervention or metformin on inflammation and coagulation in participants with impaired glucose tolerance. *Diabetes* 54 (2005):1566–1572.

27. Wing RR, Hamman RF, Bray GA, et al. Achieving weight and activity goals among diabetes prevention program lifestyle participants. *Obes Res* 12 (2004):1426–1434.

28. Laliberte R, Byers Kraus V, Rooks D. (2004). *The Everyday Arthritis Solution: Food, Movement, and Lifestyle Secrets to Ease the Pain and Feel Your Best!* (Paperback ed.). Pleasantville, NY: Reader's Digest, Inc.

29. Rooks DS, Kiel DP, Parsons C, et al. Self-paced resistance training and walking exercise in community-dwelling older adults: Effects on neuromotor performance. *J Gerontol A Biol Sci Med Sci* 52 (1997):161–168.

9

Exercise and Diabetes

Jacqueline Shahar and Osama Hamdy

Diabetes, historically, dates back to the ancient times in several cultures in the world. The Ebers Papyrus written in 1550 BCE and named after Georg Ebers, a German Egyptologist, is the first document that mentioned diabetes.[1] Hippocrates, a Greek physician, also mentioned excessive urinary flow; however, he emphasized the effect of diet, exercise, and lifestyle change as preventive medicine. Around 1000 AD, Greek physicians prescribed exercise on horseback as a way to manage diabetes and decrease excess urination.[2]

In 1857, Claude Bernard linked diabetes with glycogen metabolism, which led to the observation that the liver is a very important organ in diabetes. It was soon after this that the role of the pancreas in diabetes was found. In 1869, a German medical student, Paul Langerhans, discovered the islet cells in the pancreas, which was eventually named for him, islets of Langerhans. Twenty years later, in 1889, Joseph von Mehring and Oskar Minkowski found that dogs developed diabetes after their pancreas were removed.[2]

Frederick Banting, from the University of Toronto, and Charles Herbert discovered insulin in 1923. At that time, the approach for the treatment of diabetes was starvation (400–600 calories a day). This approach was developed by an American diabetologist, Frederick Allen.[2]

In the early 1980s human insulin became available. People with diabetes started living longer with the use of insulin, however, insulin does not cure diabetes. In fact, as the people started living longer, they developed complications including heart disease, stroke, kidney failure, amputations, and blindness. Dr. Elliot P. Joslin, in the 1930s, believed that a team approach was necessary for the management of diabetes and the prevention of those serious complications. Dr. Joslin's therapeutic approach included the education of patients in foot care, medical nutrition therapy, exercise, and treatment of foot infections. He emphasized that insulin was not a cure all for diabetes.[1] It was around this time that exercise for people with diabetes took on a greater role.

According to 2002 death certificates, diabetes was the sixth leading cause of death in the United States. As of 2005 over 14 million people in the

United States were diagnosed with diabetes, where an additional 6 million were suggested to be undiagnosed, representing 6 percent of the population. These numbers are alarming, and as staggering as these values are is the suggested total disease cost that exceeds over 130 billion dollars. A recent report suggests that one out of every eight health care dollars goes to costs due to diabetes.

Diabetes mellitus is a group of diseases that affect metabolism resulting from defects in insulin production, insulin action, or both. It is associated with hyperglycemia (high blood glucose) and hypoglycemia (low blood glucose levels) due to the body's inability to control blood glucose. Glucose is the nervous system's sole energy source and working muscles' primary fuel during exercise and physical activity. Therefore, control over glucose is vital. Insulin is a hormone secreted by the beta cells of the pancreas. It facilitates the transport of glucose across cells membranes as well as stimulates the breakdown of glycogen (the storage form of glucose). Type 1 diabetes is caused by the autoimmune destruction of the beta cells. People with Type 1 diabetes are usually dependent on insulin injections. Type 2 diabetes is caused by insulin resistance. The cells are unable to properly utilize insulin. So the pancreas produces more insulin to overcome the insulin resistance. Ultimately the pancreas cannot produce more insulin to the point that the person is diagnosed with Type 2 diabetes. Approximately 90–95 percent of people diagnosed with diabetes have Type 2. People with Type 2 diabetes are usually overweight with an excessive amount of abdominal fat, regardless of the total amount of fat. Unlike Type 1, Type 2 is associated with elevated insulin concentrations and responds to diet modification and exercise in controlling blood glucose.[3]

Diabetes is a brutal disease affecting many parts of the body, which may cause serious life-altering problems such as kidney damage, blindness, loss of sensation in fingers and toes, and limb amputations. The good news is that it can be prevented or controlled through lifestyle practices that control blood glucose, decrease body weight and body fat, and lower blood fats and blood pressure.

Alarmingly, the rate of diabetes is increasing. Between 1997 and 2002 it has increased over 40 percent. As the problem of obesity and its associated problems continue to grow, experts suggest that diabetes will increase in the future. If people do not get enough exercise and eat healthier food, they are more likely to become overweight and obese. This places them at a higher risk of getting Type 2 diabetes. Exercise has been shown to decrease body fat and weight. Exercise and increased physical activity need to become a priority for those with and without diabetes, but it has not. Only 39 percent of people with diabetes reported that they were physically active compared with 58 percent of people without diabetes in a 2003 survey by Morrato et al. They found that the proportion of active adults without diabetes declined as the number of risk factors increased until becoming similar to people with diabetes.[4] The management priority for people with diabetes is glucose control and weight loss, which can be achieved through healthy eating, medications, and exercise. The American College of Sports Medicine (ACSM) suggests that intensive treatment to control blood glucose has been documented to reduce the risk of progression of diabetic complications 50 to 75 percent in adults with Type 1 diabetes and has been considered to be of similar efficacy in adults with Type 2 diabetes. The ACSM suggests that exercise is effective in glucose control because exercise has an insulin-like effect that enhances the uptake of glucose even in the presence of insulin deficiency. The result of exercise treatment that are specific to diabetics includes improved glucose tolerance, increased insulin sensitivity, and deceased insulin and diabetes pills requirements, as well as improved lipid profiles, decreased blood pressure, weight loss, weight control, and increased physical capacity.[3]

There seems to be no single strategy in the treatment of diabetes. There are several drugs and other strategies to control prediabetes and diabetes, but again no single approach works for all people. In a 2007 meta-analyses (an analysis of many trials and studies) lifestyle interventions seemed to be at least as effective as drug therapy in preventing or delaying the progression to diabetes among people with prediabetes (impaired glucose tolerance).[5] Kim and colleagues suggested that people with Type 2 diabetes who followed lifestyle changes, including a healthy diet and increased physical activity, may improve the early signs of cardiovascular disease, such as decreasing in carotid intima-media thickness (IMT) and blood pressure.[6] This is good news because more than 65 percent of people with diabetes die from heart disease and stroke. These lifestyle changes can be started by most people, take a little bit of time, can be free of charge, and most importantly have a wide range of health benefits.

So for those with prediabetes or those who have it, the question of should I exercise has been answered and the question of how should I exercise should be asked.

WHAT HAPPENS DURING EXERCISE?

Several metabolic, hormonal, and cardiovascular changes occur in your body during exercise. The carbohydrates that you eat get stored in the liver and in muscles as glycogen. What you eat also contains fat, which gets stored as triglycerides in fat tissue. During exercise, you move your leg and arm muscles. Your heart is pumping at a faster rate, blood pressure and blood flow increases to the active muscles. Initially, these muscles utilize stored energy without the use of oxygen. As you continue to exercise, oxygen supply becomes available to break down carbohydrates, fat, and protein to be used as energy for the continuous exercise. After approximately five to ten minutes, the liver becomes the main energy source for the active muscles and produces glucose. Glycogen stores in the muscles are depleted after about twenty to thirty minutes of continuous exercise. Free fatty acids (stored triglycerides in fat tissue) are utilized in addition to the break down of glucose by the liver.[7]

Your muscles contract with exercise. Exercise causes the activation of glucose transport by GLUT 4. The protein carrier, GLUT 4, helps increase glucose uptake by the active muscles. As the frequency and duration of exercise increases, the number of GLUT 4 that are available to move more glucose to the active muscle increase as well.[8]

Your body also secrets counterregulatory hormones (epinephrine, norepinephrine, growth hormone, and cortisol) that help maintaining blood glucose level as you exercise. Insulin secretion is reduced to facilitate production of glucose by the liver. Glucagon is also released to increase glucose production by the liver and glucose in the blood stream. In people with Type 1 diabetes, insulin secretion is not reduced because it is delivered by injection. Glucose production by the liver remains low, therefore, the risk for hypoglycemia is significant. At a moderate intensity of exercise, your body will utilize about 50 percent of the energy needed from carbohydrates. However, at a very high intensity of exercise, most of the energy used by your muscles will come from carbohydrates. The counterregulatory hormones signal the liver to produce more glucose from glycogen stores that may exceed the amount of required energy, therefore at the end of your exercise session blood glucose value will be higher than pre exercise session.[9]

As you finish your exercise session, your muscles will recover themselves by continuously utilizing glucose twenty-four to forty-eight hours after the exercise session is completed. This means that blood glucose will continue decreasing. In people who inject insulin or take curtain diabetes pills (see Insulin and Diabetes Pills section), concentration of insulin is not reduced. This can increase glucose utilization that can lead to hypoglycemia.[8,9] See Precautions and Guidelines for Management of Blood Glucose with Exercise.

DIAGNOSIS

Diabetes is a group of metabolic diseases involving abnormal glucose levels associated with several acute and chronic complications.[10] It is characterized by hyperglycemia (high blood glucose), which results from problems with the release of insulin from the pancreas, the action of insulin, or both.[11]

Diabetes is diagnosed by checking fasting (no food for at least eight hours) glucose levels. One would be diagnosed with diabetes if the fasting glucose level is greater than or equal to 126mg/dl confirmed by repeated tests. With only one test, this glucose level is considered a provisional diagnosis of diabetes. Normal fasting glucose levels should be less than 100mg/dl (5.6mmol/l). Impaired fasting glucose (IFG) involves a fasting glucose level between 100mg/dl (5.6mmol/l) and 125mg/dl (6.9mmol/l).[11]

Another way to diagnose diabetes is with an Oral Glucose Tolerance Test (OGTT). This test involves drinking 75g of glucose dissolved in water and checking glucose levels after two hours. If the glucose level is greater than or equal to 140mg/dl (7.8mmol/l) but less than 200mg/dl (11.1mmol/l), the person has impaired glucose tolerance (IGT). A provisional diagnosis of diabetes is made if the glucose level is greater than 200mg/dl. A diagnosis of diabetes will be determined if the person has a glucose level greater than 200mg/dl along with classic symptoms of diabetes such as polyuria (excess urination), polydipsia (increased thirst sensation), and unexplained weight loss.[11]

BARRIERS TO EXERCISE

If you are not active and struggle with starting to exercise or being compliant with exercise, you should identify what are your barriers. It is not always easy to stick to a regular exercise schedule. Many potential obstacles can stand in the way. The following barriers are common for people with and without diabetes.

1. Lack of time—not having enough time is the number one barrier. Put exercise at high priority. Schedule at least ten- to twenty-minute time slots that can be used for planned exercise.
2. Social influence—not having support from people around you makes exercise more difficult. Get support from family and friends. Plan your social activities around exercise, make new friends that like to exercise, or join an exercise group such as mall walking.
3. Lack of energy—not having energy limits your physical movement. Exercise will help increase your blood flow and oxygen consumption, which can increase your energy level. Try to find times during the day when you feel more energetic and exercise during these times. This will help get you more energy over time.
4. Lack of will power/motivation—you might find exercise boring and not enjoyable. Choose fun and easy activities that require minimal preparation, such as walking on a treadmill or cycling on a stationary bike while watching a show or listening to music.
5. Fear of injury—you are afraid of injuring your knee, back, etc. To avoid injury, start with an exercise that you feel confident doing or that you have some experience doing, such as walking or biking. Hire a personal trainer to teach you the proper form of a variety of exercises. Start your exercise session with a warm up and end it with a cool down and progress slowly. Wear comfortable walking shoes. In order to know what type of walking shoes you need, do a search on line, find information from running magazines, or go to a specialized running shoe store to evaluate your walking gait and match the appropriate shoe for you.
6. Lack of skills—choose activities with familiar skills, such as walking, biking, or taking stairs. To learn new skills, join a class or hire a personal trainer.
7. Lack of resources—you may live or work in a city where health clubs, bike trails, or safe areas to exercise are not nearby. In addition, it can be too cold, too hot or humid, or the sidewalks are not clear so you cannot exercise safely outside. These restrictions reduce the chance that you will be physically active. Fortunately, there are alternatives: join a health club located on the way to or from work or buy home exercise equipment, such as exercise tapes/DVDs, treadmill, stationary bike, elliptical machine, cross trainer, arm

ergometer, free weights, stretching bands, physioball, or other devices. These are great choices to be physically active.[12]

Now you can identify which barriers apply to you. If you have more than one barrier, start working on the barrier that is easiest for you to change. Once you have succeeded with that barrier, you can move on to the next one. By implementing these solutions, you can become physically active.

HEALTH BENEFITS OF EXERCISE FOR PEOPLE AT RISK OF DEVELOPING OR HAVING DIABETES

Regular and long-term exercise provides many benefits for a person who wants to prevent or has diabetes. These benefits are both physiological and psychological and include the following:

1. Improves glycemic control. Glucose is an energy source for your muscles. With exercise muscles contract and require more glucose. The more muscles you move during exercise, the more glucose you will use. This will help improve glycemic control.[13] Several studies have shown that supervised weight training is a good way to control Type 2 diabetes. One supervised study found high-intensity progressive resistance training, in combination with moderate weight loss, increased strength and lean body mass and was effective in improving glycemic control in older patients with Type 2 diabetes.[14] Dunstan et al. also found that center-based, supervised but not home-based resistance training was associated with the maintenance of modestly improved glycemic control in subjects who started an initial laboratory-supervised resistance training program. Unfortunately, the people in the at-home program did not follow their program as well and, therefore, did not show any long-term improvements in blood glucose control and insulin sensitivity. Exercise should be a key part of all people's lifestyles, especially among those who have diabetes. As these researchers pointed out, sticking to home exercise programs is a major challenge for most people, with and without diabetes. They pointed to the importance of resistance training for people who have diabetes, along with the need of supervised exercise programs.[15]
2. Increases metabolism and promotes weight loss. Exercise helps strengthen and build your muscles. An increase in muscle mass helps burn more calories and promotes weight loss.[13] This is correlated with a reduction in waist circumference.[16] Waist circumference is an important marker because increased intra-abdominal fat has been associated most closely with metabolic abnormalities.[17]
3. Reduces risk of metabolic syndrome by 41 percent and reduces the risk of developing diabetes by 58 percent.[13] The metabolic syndrome is a group of risk factors that can lead to Type 2 diabetes. These risks factors include: high blood pressure, abdominal obesity, hyperglycemia, high triglycerides, and low level of HDL cholesterol.[18]
4. Improves insulin sensitivity. Insulin works better as a result of exercising.[8] This can decrease the amount of insulin or diabetes pills you take. Exercising

at more than 70 percent of maximum heart rate 150–200 minutes per week will have stronger effect on insulin sensitivity and reduce the risk of metabolic syndrome.[16]

5. Improves blood pressure. Exercise results in a decrease of 5 to 10mmHg in systolic and diastolic blood pressure.[8]
6. Reduces risk factors of heart disease. Exercise reduces your bad (LDL) cholesterol and triglycerides and increases your good (HDL) cholesterol.[8] This reduction is important because Type 2 diabetes often leads to cardiovascular disease, which causes heart attacks and strokes. More than 65 percent of people with diabetes die from heart disease and strokes.[19] Not all people are able to do strenuous exercise. For many, walking, such as mall walking, is what they can tolerate. Fritz and associates found that people with diabetes who performed normal walking three days a week for forty-five minutes improved blood pressure, body mass index, and cholesterol levels in the their blood. Even though these values were improved, the ability to handle glucose and insulin were not. The researchers suggested that exercise intensity was not measured and could have been too low to have an effect on blood glucose.[20] The ACSM suggests walking may be the activity of choice for many people for it is readily accessible, offers tolerable exercise intensity, and is easily regulated. Brisk walking (2.9–3.9 mph), which is a moderate intensity for most people, has also been shown to increase aerobic capacity and decrease body weight and body fat in previously sedentary middle-aged men.
7. Reduces stress.[21]
8. Reduces depression and improves well-being.[21]
9. Enhances independent activity of daily living.[21]
10. Increases muscular strength and tone of muscles.[13]
11. Improves flexibility.[13]
12. Improves cardio respiratory fitness.[21] Cardio respiratory fitness of moderate to high levels and muscular strength help prevent diabetes.[16] Working on your fitness may be more important than working on your weight. Lee and associates found that men who had a higher cardio respiratory fitness had a lower chance of getting the precursors related to diabetes, even if they were overweight. The relative risks of having the metabolic syndrome were 1.8 and 1.6 times higher in the low and moderate cardio respiratory fitness groups, compared with the high-cardio respiratory fitness group after adjusting for age, visceral fat, and subcutaneous fat.[22] This doesn't mean bringing bodyweight to an acceptable range is not recommended, it is highly, we only are illustrating the importance of exercise and increasing ones fitness level.
13. Reduces the need for diabetes medication.[7]
14. Increases bone density.[21]
15. Attenuates the progression of peripheral neuropathy in people with diabetes who have it. Peripheral neuropathy is a common complication of diabetes and can often lead to amputation. Diabetes, according to Balducci et al., is the major cause of peripheral neuropathy and no definitive treatment for the neuropathy has been established. Balducci found that long-term aerobic exercise training could prevent the onset or modify the natural history of peripheral neuropathy.[23]

16. Reduces health care cost. A 2005 research study reported by the American Diabetes Association found that inactive people with Type 2 diabetes who walked three miles or more every day were in better health and had lower medical expenses after two years, while their sedentary counterparts had higher healthcare costs and diminished health. Even though weight was not lost individuals who exercised thirty-eight minutes per day lowered their blood pressure, cholesterol, AIC levels, and heart disease risk. The increase in activity equaled about 2,200 extra steps a day, which is not a considerable amount of time to reap such important health changes and you can even say financial benefits.[24]

HEALTH BENEFITS OF PHYSICAL ACTIVITY

People trying to manage their diabetes should not just exercise; they should try to increase daily physical activity as well. Physical activity is different from formal exercise. It refers to daily routines that increase energy demands, such as walking the dog, taking the stairs instead of the elevator, or walking a greater distance from your car to a building's entrance. Sometimes increasing physical activity is all that people can fit into their lives. Hu and colleagues found that people with Type 2 diabetes who were physically active at moderate to high intensity had a reduced risk of total and cardiovascular mortality, regardless of the levels of body mass index, blood pressure, total cholesterol, and smoking.[20] Kim and colleagues supported the importance of increased physical activity. They suggested that people with Type 2 diabetes who followed lifestyle changes including a healthy diet and increased level of physical activity appeared to improve the early symptoms of cardiovascular disease.[25]

TESTING

The ACSM suggests prior to starting an exercise program, people with diabetes should undergo an extensive medical evaluation particularly for the cardiovascular, nervous, renal, and visual systems because they are related to diabetic complications. Simple cardiovascular tests of resting heart rate (tachycardia) as well as heart rate and blood pressure response to an orthostatic challenge (a fall in systolic blood pressure >20 mmHg upon standing), deep breathing, and Valsalva maneuver (breath holding against a closed glottis) can provide information on the extent of autonomic neuropathy.[3]

Because people with diabetes are at higher risk for heart disease, they should always check with their physicians before undertaking vigorous exercise. People with diabetes should be assessed for conditions that might be associated with the increased probability of coronary vascular disease or that might contraindicate certain types of exercise or predispose to injury. Also, people who start moderate to vigorous exercise (more than brisk walking) need to have a graded exercise test (GXT). The GXT is used to assess cardio respiratory function.[26]

A GXT consists of walking on a treadmill at increasing speeds and inclines. This is performed until you reach your maximum tolerance. You are monitored for cardio respiratory functioning, which consists of ECG, blood pressure, heart rate, oxygen uptake, breathing frequency, and other variables.[26] Imaging of the heart using echocardiography at rest and during exercise can increase the accuracy of the test. Exercise nuclear imaging using thallium or technetium is used to show the amount of blood supply in areas of the heart. Reduced blood supply indicates a problem.[21]

A pharmacological stress test is used with people who have orthopedic problems that limit walking on a treadmill, peripheral vascular disease (PVD), very poor exercise capacity, and neurological disease. Injection of Dobutamine will increase heart rate and oxygen demand that may show heart abnormality. Dipridamole or adenosine injections show flow of blood in the areas of the heart. Use of imaging is helpful when diagnosis cannot be confirmed only by GXT.[21]

The following criteria are used to decide who needs to have a GXT.[21]

1. Any person with diabetes above age of 35.
2. Any person with diabetes above age of 25 with more than ten years duration of Type 2 diabetes or more than fifteen years duration of Type 1 diabetes.
3. Any person with diabetes with additional heart disease risk factors, such as:
   - Obesity—BMI of $30kg/m^2$ or waist circumference of 40 inches (102 cm) or more in men and 35 inches (88 cm) or more in women. Excessive fat in the abdomen (apple shape) increases the risk for coronary artery disease.
   - Tobacco—Current cigarette smoker or someone who quit smoking in the past six months. Cigarette smoking and the use of other tobacco is hazardous and increases the risk for heart disease, as well as those who already had a coronary event or revascularization procedure.
   - Hypertension—Hypertension increases stress on the heart muscle and can lead to injury of the heart. Having one of the following on two separate occasions would indicate a risk factor:
     - Systolic blood pressure of 140mmHg or above
     - Diastolic blood pressure of 90mmHg or above
   - Family history—having a father or first degree relative (brother or son) who had a heart attack, revascularization, or died before the age of 55 or a mother or first degree relative (sister or daughter) who had a heart attack, revascularization, or died before the age of 65 increases the risk for coronary heart disease.
   - Physical inactivity—Not participating in an exercise program or not doing leisure time physical activity increases the risk for cardiovascular artery disease.
   - High cholesterol—Having one of the following is considered as a risk factor for heart disease:
     - Total cholesterol of 200mg/dl (5.2mmol/L) or above. There is a positive and continuous relationship between total cholesterol level and mortality rate.

- LDL cholesterol of 130mg/dl (3.4mmol/L) or above. LDL cholesterol damages the walls of arteries in the body.
- HDL cholesterol below 35mg/dl (0.9mmol/L). HDL cholesterol removes the bad (LDL) cholesterol from the arteries. For every 1mg/dl of increase in HDL cholesterol, there is a 2–3 percent reduction in risk for coronary heart disease.[21,27]

4. Anyone having microvascular disease: eye disease (proliferative diabetic retinopathy), kidney disease (nephropathy).
5. Anyone having peripheral vascular disease (PAD). PAD is very common in people with diabetes and can lead to heart and blood vessel disease.
6. Anyone having autonomic neuropathy. Autonomic neuropathy is a complication of diabetes that causes damage to the nerves. There is a miscommunication between the brain and nerves in your body, which reduces the ability to sense when becoming hypoglycemic or having problems in the heart such as heart attack. Autonomic neuropathy is manifested by abnormal heart rate, orthostatic hypotension, gastrointestinal symptoms such as, nausea, vomiting, constipation, trouble in digestion and urination, and sexual difficulties.[28]

EXERCISE PRESCRIPTION

For the most part, those who are young and have their blood glucose under control can participate in a variety of activities. Those who are middle aged and older should consider activities that are low impact on their bones and joints. As with anyone who is older, especially people with diabetes, before initiating an exercise program a medical evaluation is warranted.[3]

Prescribing an exercise plan involves many different components. These include the specific type of exercise (mode), how hard you will exercise (intensity), how long (duration), how many times per week (frequency), and how you will progress. The components of any training session should include a warm up and cool down.

SYMPTOMS OF HYPOGLYCEMIA AND HYPERGLYCEMIA

Two important exercise considerations for people with diabetes are hypoglycemia and hyperglycemia. The ACSM suggests that hypoglycemia is the most common problem for diabetics who exercise. Exercise and daily physical activity can lower your blood glucose below normal levels, causing hypoglycemia, especially in people who take insulin or certain anti diabetic oral medications. It can happen during exercise, just afterwards, or even up to twenty-four to forty-eight hours later. Symptoms of hypoglycemia involve disruption in motor and mental function, which is called nueroglycopenia.[29] Hyperglycemia can be associated with exercise. See Table 9.1 with the list of symptoms for hypoglycemia and hyperglycemia that are the same for people with Type 1 and Type 2 diabetes.[7]

Some people with diabetes need to avoid certain kinds of physical activity due to complications such as high blood pressure, peripheral neuropathy,

Table 9.1
Symptoms for Hypoglycemia and Hyperglycemia That Are the Same for People with Type 1 and Type 2 Diabetes

Hyperglycemia (High Sugar) Symptoms	Hypoglycemia (Low Sugar) Symptoms
Increase thirst	Shaking/trembling
Increase hunger	Sweating
Increase fatigue, weakness, malaise	Hunger, nausea
Increase urination	Weakness
Blurred vision	Headache, dizziness
Deep, rapid breathing not relate to exertion (kussmaul respiration)	Confusion, slow thinking, slurred speech, trouble concentrating
Headache	Fatigue/sleepiness
Nausea, vomiting, abdominal pain	Blurred vision
Weight loss	Fast pulse, pounding heart
No symptoms	Tingling in extremities
	Heavy breathing
	No coordination
	No symptoms

retinopathy, autonomic neuropathy, foot infection, and peripheral vascular disease. See the Precautions section for guidelines before you start exercising.

EXERCISE MODES—THE MOST COMMON AND USEFUL

Exercise mode refers to the specific activity done by people with diabetes. Activities that use major muscles groups over a long period of time are aerobic exercise.[9] Resistance training also called weight training involves exercising using resistance in the form of free weights, stretching bands, or machines. The last type of exercise is flexibility exercise, which is also called stretching.[4]

Aerobic Exercise

Aerobic exercise needs to done for a minimum of thirty minutes up to ninety minutes of continuous exercise if weight loss and avoiding regain is the goal.[3,30] However, you can also exercise intermittently for ten minutes several times during the day. Aerobic exercise promotes the development and maintenance of cardiovascular health. This includes reducing risk factors of heart disease, decreasing blood pressure and bad cholesterol, and increasing good cholesterol and cardio respiratory fitness. Aerobic exercise includes walking, cycling, swimming, water exercise, dancing, and the use of aerobic machines, such as elliptical, Airdyne bike, recumbent bike, arm ergometer, Nu Step, treadmill, stair stepper, and rowing. Other ways you can improve your endurance is through cross and interval training.[21]

Cross training involves alternating exercises such as walking, cycling, rowing, swimming, arm bike, weight training, aerobic classes, yoga, and other exercises over different days. This adds variety and flexibility to your exercise program, which can decrease boredom. Cross training helps reduce the risk of injury by distributing the physical stress of training to different muscles.[31] Choose a variety of activities that you enjoy and include all of them in your exercise program rather than just having a single activity. With cross training, you will be able to avoid injury, stay motivated, and achieve significant results.

Interval training involves doing aerobic exercise for intervals at a higher intensity than you would normally do. Each interval can last 60–120 seconds or longer, with similar time for rest intervals. This training should be performed after you have already established a basic level of endurance and strength.[31] Interval training can help reduce hemoglobin A1c and assist with the management of diabetes.[32] With interval training you burn more calories than continuous aerobic training, which makes weight loss somewhat easier. Interval training helps make the exercise session go by faster. In a study done by Arnt E. Tjonna, interval training was compared to a continuous moderate intensity aerobic exercise in people with metabolic syndrome. Interval training was done four times for four minutes each at 90–95 percent of maximum heart rate, with three minutes recovery at 70 percent of maximum heart rate. The continuous aerobic exercise was done at 70 percent of maximum heart rate for forty-seven minutes. Tjonna found that people who performed the high intensity interval training were able to significantly reduce metabolic syndrome risk factors.[33]

An example of interval training is that you spend three to five minutes warming up at an easy pace for you. Change your speed/intensity every minute. Walk at a speed of 3.0 mph for one minute. Increase your speed to 3.5 mph or increase the incline to 3 percent for one minute, and then reduce your speed back to 3.0 mph. At the end, spend three to five minutes cooling down at an easy pace. Many cardiovascular machines such as treadmills, bikes, cross trainers, and ellipticals have built-in interval programs. However, you can create your own interval training that works best for you following the example above. You should establish basic level of endurance before you try interval training.

Resistance Training

Resistance training uses free weights, weight machines, or stretching bands to increase muscle strength or endurance. With age, you lose muscle tissue and gain fat, which leads to a reduction of energy metabolism.[13] Resistance training helps promote weight loss by increasing your muscle mass, which increases your metabolism. Other health benefits from resistance training include an increase in bone density that helps avoid osteoporosis and an increase in muscle mass and muscle tone that increase self-image. It improves activity of daily living and reduces the risk of injury. As your muscles get stronger, your daily activities such as taking the stairs or getting up from sitting on a chair will be easier to perform. People with diabetes may have joint pain as a result of being overweight or playing sports. Doing resistance exercises that target major muscle groups such as the legs, trunk, and arms helps with reducing stress on the ankles, knees, or lower back, which will reduce the risk for injury.[13] More research on the effects of resistance exercise on diabetes is progressing, more is needed, but what has been done so far has shown beneficial effects such as improvements in blood glucose control and insulin sensitivity.[34]

With any type of resistance exercise, you should start with a warm up and end the activity with a cool down. Select eight to ten exercises that target major muscle groups. Learn the proper form for each exercise and do one set of ten to twelve repetitions. Slowly progress to two sets of fifteen repetitions. It is important not to hold your breath while doing the exercises. Remember to breathe out during the exertion. You can start with 2lbs weights or light resistance stretching band, and you should feel exertion during the last two to three repetitions of each set. Perform each movement in a slow manner. Count to three when performing the movement, as well as when returning to the starting position. Rest for one or two minutes between sets if doing exercises at a higher intensity or lifting a heavier weight.[7,13,34] However, if you do resistance exercises at a lower intensity or using less weight, your rest time should be less than thirty seconds. This will keep your heart rate elevated and provide some cardio respiratory benefits.

Many people with diabetes, especially those who are just starting, should follow the ACSM guidelines.

The ACSM resistance training prescription emphasizes using lower resistance.

Intensity: 40–60 percent of one repetition maximum (1 RM) and lower intensity (avoiding momentary muscular failure) is recommended. 1 RM is the maximum amount that you can lift in one repetition. The ACSM suggests healthy adults to achieve momentary muscular failure when resistance training, but not those who have diabetes.

Duration: One set of exercises for the major muscle groups with ten to fifteen repetitions; progress to fifteen to twenty.

Frequency: The minimum frequency is two per week, with at least forty-eight hours in between sessions.

Proper technique, including minimizing sustained gripping, static work, and the Valsalva maneuver (breath holding against a closed glottis) is essential to prevent a hypertensive response.

Stretching Exercise

Stretching exercise involves loosening up your muscles to prevent them from tightening or cramping after doing resistance or aerobic exercise. Muscles tighten up following exercise, which can cause pain or reduce the range of motion. Therefore, it is imperative to stretch your muscles after you exercise or when your muscles are warm. Stretching will increase range of motion and help avoid joint and muscle pain.[4] Hold a specific muscle or muscle group in a stretched position for fifteen to thirty seconds. Each muscle group should be stretched two to four times for optimal results. This is called static stretching. It requires little time or assistance, is effective, and has a low risk of injury.[21]

Yoga can also be used to help stretch muscles. However, one should only start performing yoga with an experienced yoga instructor. The stretching techniques of yoga may help patients with Type 2 diabetes reduce their need for oral antidiabetic medications, as well as lower cholesterol and blood pressure.[35]

Intensity of Exercise

There are several different options to determine your exercise intensity, which involves how hard the exercise feels like. These options are based on the guidelines of the American College of Sports Medicine.[21]

The specific ACSM cardio respiratory exercise guidelines for people with diabetes are:

Frequency: three to four days a week and progress to five days a week
Duration: twenty to sixty minutes
Intensity: 50–80 percent of heart rate reserve (HRR) or 70–89 percent of maximal heart rate

The ACSM recommends using 40 percent to 85 percent of heart rate reserve (HRR) or 64 percent to 94 percent of maximum heart rate when prescribing exercise to most healthy adults, while 50 to 80 percent of HRR or 70 to 89 percent of maximal heart rate for people with diabetes. This wide range is not appropriate for all. Heart rate ranges should differ based on level of initial condition, especially in the deconditioned. A recent report suggested that exercising at 70 percent or more of maximum heart rate will have a stronger effect on insulin sensitivity. This corresponds to exercising at 50 percent or more of HRR or a rating of perceived exertion of moderate to somewhat hard.[16]

Since most people do not know their *maximum heart rate*, it is easiest to calculate using the following option. To calculate maximum heart rate, take 220 minus your age. Then calculate 50 percent to 80 percent of this value to determine your heart rate range while exercising. For example, a 40 year old would have a maximum heart rate of 180. The 40 year old should therefore exercise with a heart rate range of 90 to 144 beats per minute (bpm). Unfit or sedentary people should start exercising at 50 percent to 60 percent of maximum HR.

Exercise professionals prefer to use the HRR versus the maximum heart rate percent method. HRR is the difference between the maximum heart rate and resting heart rate. In the percent HRR method, a percentage of heart rate reserve is added to the resting heart rate to determine the target heart rate.

Heart rate = {% exercise intensity × (HR max − HR rest)} × HR rest.

Example: A male, aged 40, with a resting heart rate of 60, who wants to train at 50 to 85 percent of HRR will be as follows:

$$HR = [.50 \times \{(220 - 40) - 60\}] + 60 = 120$$

$$HR = [.85 \times \{(220 - 40) - 60\}] + 60 = 162$$

Therefore, the target heart rate range is 120 to 162 bpm.

Most people can safely exercise within a target heart rate range. However, beginners generally do better at the lower end of the range (less intense exercise to start). Additionally, people who are on medications to control blood pressure (antihypertensive medication) may not have an increase in heart rate the way that they would without the medication. Therefore, if you are on medications to control blood pressure, you need to consult with your doctor before determining your exercise heart range and you should use the Rating of Perceived Exertion (RPE) to judge the exercise intensity.

The maximum heart rate formula (Max heart rate = 220 − age) is not entirely accurate due to a plus or minus 20 beat error of estimate; in other words 95 percent of 40-year-old men and women have a maximum heart rate between 160 and 200 beats/min. This shows that predicted maximum heart rate values as well as training ranges determined from it have a high degree of error associated with them. We are not saying not to use it, but we recommend a combination of RPE and heart rate when monitoring the intensity of aerobic exercise.[21]

The RPE scale is a useful tool to measure intensity of exercise. This scale correlates well with heart rate and workload and is used for people who have difficulty measuring their own HR or taking medication that affect their heart rate. As you exercise, subjectively rate the exertion of your activity. The scale is from 0–10. A 0 means that the exertion is "nothing at all," and 10 is "extremely strong." See Table 9.2 for the RPE scale. Generally, you should exercise at a level between 3 and 5.[21]

The Talk Test can also be used to measure intensity of exercise. If you can whistle or sing while exercising, the intensity is low and you should speed up or increase the resistance. If you can carry a conversation, but not whistle while exercising, the intensity is considered moderate. This is the suggested intensity at which you should exercise. If you are short of breath, the intensity is so vigorous that you should slow down or reduce the resistance. You should stop exercising if you have chest discomfort or any joint or muscle pain.[36,37]

Frequency of Exercise

This depends on the mode of exercise and what your goals are. Aerobic exercise can be performed for at least thirty minutes that can be done intermittently (minimum of ten-minutes bouts in a day), at least three to four days

Table 9.2
RPE Scale

0	Nothing at all
0.5	Extremely weak
1	Very Weak
2	Weak
3	Moderate
4	
5	Strong
6	
7	Very strong
8	
9	
10	Extremely strong

a week. Interval training should be done at most one to two times per week. Resistance exercise should be performed at least two days a week with one day of rest in between. Stretching can be performed daily.[3,21,34]

The ACSM suggests that people with Type 2 diabetes should strive to accumulate a minimum of 1,000 kcal per week of physical activity. Greater amounts of caloric expenditure (2,000 kcal per week), including daily exercise, may be required if weight loss is a goal.

Warm Up

Warm up is the first five to ten minutes of the exercise session, which helps the body adjust from rest to exercise. It increases body temperature and blood flow and as a result helps avoid musculoskeletal injury. In addition, the warm up phase decreases the risk for irregular heart rhythm. An example for warm up on a treadmill is to start at 2.0–2.3 mph and progress to 3.0–3.5 mph after five to ten minutes. Then continue at this speed for forty minutes (endurance phase). The same concept can be applied if walking outside, biking, or using any cardio/aerobic machine.[21]

Cool Down

Cool down is the last five to ten minutes of the exercise session, which helps the working muscles recover. Heart rate and blood pressure return to near resting values, which results in preventing dizziness and low blood pressure post exercise. The cool down also facilitates the removal of lactic acid from working muscles. An example of a cool down if you were walking on a treadmill at 3.5 mph is to reduce the speed slowly to 2.0–2.3 mph or less over the last five to ten minutes and then stop the treadmill.[21]

Tools and Equipment

Many options of aerobic machines can help you improve cardio respiratory system function and stamina. Treadmills, bikes, and elliptical machines target your leg muscles only, however, cross trainers, Airdynes, rowing, and Nu Step machines target both your legs and arms. Nonweight-bearing activities, such as water aerobics, swimming, or any sitting aerobic machine, such as a recumbent bike, upright bike, Nu Step, Airdyne, can be used to avoid additional stress on the joints. Weight-bearing activities such as walking, jogging, running, or hiking can be performed if you don't have muscle skeletal problems. An arm bike can be performed if you cannot do any aerobic exercise using leg muscles or when you need to rest your leg muscles.[21]

Resistance training can be performed using free weights, resistance machines such as Cybex or Nautilus, stretching bands, or your own body weight. Nautilus and Cybex machines are used when starting a resistance exercise program in a gym. It helps you perform exercises properly and is easy to progress. Free weights can be used at home or in a gym. With free weights you use more muscles and motor units to perform the exercises appropriately. It is important to learn the correct form under supervision to avoid injury. Stretching bands are elastic bands with handles. They have different colors to correspond with different resistances. The thicker the band, the more resistance it creates on your muscles. Using stretching bands forces you to work in more controlled movements because on the return movement the band pulls you toward the starting position. You can carry the stretching bands with you when you travel, it requires very little space, it is cheaper than other resistance equipment, it is convenient to use, it allows you to do many exercises, and it can target many muscle groups. However, the bands become less elastic with use, which means they become less effective over time.[13]

INSULIN AND DIABETES PILLS

Insulin and some diabetes pills may put you at risk for hypoglycemia, especially when you exercise and do physical activity. Any type of insulin will put you at risk for hypoglycemia. To avoid hypoglycemia, you need to know what time you plan to exercise or be physically active, which insulin is working at that time and for how long, and how much of the total dosage of insulin you should reduce.

The following group of diabetes pills may put you at a higher risk for hypoglycemia. These pills include: Glyburide (Diabeta, Micronase, Glynase), Glipizide (Glucotrol, Glucotrol XL), Glymperide (Amaryl), Metformin and Glyburide (Glucovance), Metformin and Glipizide (Metaglip), Repaglinide (Prandin), Nateglinide (Starlix), Exenatide (Byetta), and Pramlitide (Symlin).

Another group of diabetes pills include Glucophage (Metformin), Avandia (Rosiglitizone), Avandamet (Metformin/Rosiglitizone), Actos (Pioglitazone),

Precose (Acarbose), and Glyset (Miglitol). If you are only taking diabetes pills listed in the second group, the risk for hypoglycemia is much lower.[38] See Guidelines section on blood glucose check with exercise/physical activity and how to avoid hypoglycemia.

Over time, as you become more active, your body will be more sensitive to the diabetes pills; you will improve your diabetes control and lose weight. Therefore, expect that your blood glucose will drop.

PRECAUTIONS

People with diabetes are at risk to develop complications. Exercise can exacerbate complications that can lead to a disability. You need to speak with your health care provider and/or a clinical exercise physiologist who is a certified diabetes educator (CDE) before you start an exercise program. Assessment of the following diabetes complications needs to be included in order to reduce the risk of cardiovascular disease and to avoid exacerbation of complications or exercise related injury:

1. Hyperglycemia or ketosis in people with Type 1 diabetes—you may be at risk for hyperglycemia and your body can produce ketones, which can lead to Diabetes KetoAcidosis (DKA) especially if your diabetes control is poor. Blood glucose values can stay high two hours after exercise session.[9,39]

2. Exercise-induced hypoglycemia—if you exercise at least every other day, your body will be more sensitive to insulin; therefore, you will improve your blood glucose control. However, you could be at risk for hypoglycemia during or after exercise. This mechanism most likely occurs due to increased utilization of glucose by the active muscles, the need to replenish the active muscles post exercise, and reduced glucose production by the liver that could last twenty-four to forty-eight hours.[9,40]

3. High blood pressure—if you have high blood pressure you should avoid vigorous activity, heavy weight lifting, and holding your breath when exercising. Aerobic activity is preferred to reduce blood pressure. Do not exercise if your systolic blood pressure is above 200mmHg or your diastolic blood pressure is above 110mmHg.[21]

4. Peripheral neuropathy—is a reduction in pain sensation in the feet, which increases the risk for skin breakdown, foot infections, and destruction of the arches in the foot (Charcot foot). A reduction in pain sensation can make it hard to distinguish if you injured your feet during exercise, which may cause additional problems if exercise continues. If you have peripheral neuropathy, avoid performing long sessions of weight-bearing activities, such as walking, hiking, or jogging. Engage in nonweight-bearing activities such as biking, swimming, arm biking, or chair resistance exercise using free weights, stretching bands, and wrist or ankle weights.[7] You can combine weight-bearing and nonweight-bearing activities. Be aware that peripheral neuropathy may result in balance and gait abnormalities during exercise. There are many exercise options to choose from that will allow you to work within your limitations.

5. Retinopathy—can be assessed by a thorough ophthalmic examination with dilated pupils. It is necessary for all people with diabetes to have an ophthalmic examination two to three months before starting an exercise plan. In the presence of moderate to severe nonproliferative diabetic retinopathy (NPDR), you should avoid heavy weight lifting or holding your breath during exercise (Valsalva maneuver).[9] With proliferative diabetic retinopathy (PDR), the risk of triggering vitreous hemorrhage or retinal detachment is high. Therefore, with PDR or macular edema avoid activities that elevate blood pressure significantly, such as heavy weight lifting, high impact aerobics, jarring activities, jogging/running, racquet sports, strenuous trumpet playing, activities with your head down (yoga, power yoga, Pilates, gymnastics), or any other vigorous activity that is part of your daily routine, such as lifting furniture or heavy shopping bags.[7]

6. Autonomic neuropathy—those with autonomic neuropathy have difficulty with thermoregulation, therefore they should be advised to avoid activity in hot or cold weather. Sudden death and silent myocardial ischemia have been linked to diabetics with autonomic neuropathy. Hypotension and hypertension after vigorous physical activity is common in patients with autonomic neuropathy, particularly when initiating a physical activity program. If you have autonomic neuropathy, your doctor must test your heart before starting any exercise program. Do not follow general heart rate guidelines because your heart may not respond to exercise in a normal way or you may experience low blood pressure when changing positions. It is recommended to use the Talk Test or RPE scale. Check blood glucose before and after activity due to the risk of hypoglycemia and avoid activity with changing positions because of the risk of hypotension.[7,21]

7. Foot infection—if you have a foot infection, keep your feet clean and dry, avoid swimming, and stay off your feet. Check your feet for sores, blisters, irritation, cuts, or other injuries after you exercise.[10]

8. Peripheral vascular disease (PVD)—if you have PVD, you may experience pain mostly in your lower legs because of reduced oxygen supply to active muscles in that area. Walking intervals at low to moderate intensity with rest periods can help increase circulation of blood to active muscles in your lower legs. However, avoid walking if you feel pain at rest or at night.[7]

9. Nephropathy—people with diabetes who have nephropathy (kidney disease) often have a reduced exercise capacity. It is preferred to engage in low to moderate exercise and avoid strenuous activity, unless blood pressure is monitored.[7]

10. Worsening of diabetes complications—check with your health care provider or a CDE if any of your diabetes complications get worse and whether or not you can exercise.[7]

GUIDELINES TO BE FOLLOWED FOR ALL PEOPLE WITH DIABETES

1. Check your blood glucose before and after the exercise session. It is also recommended to check your blood glucose half way through the exercise session to gather data and learn the impact of different types of exercise and

any physical activities (house cleaning, painting, vacuuming, mowing the lawn, yard work, shopping, etc.) on your blood glucose in order to improve glucose control.

- If you take insulin or certain diabetes pills (see Insulin and Diabetes Pills section), you are at risk for hypoglycemia during and after exercise/physical activity. If you are on insulin and your blood glucose before or after the exercise session/physical activity is below 110mg/dl, you should ingest 15–30 grams of carbohydrates.[7,9]
- If you are on diabetes pills that put you at risk for hypoglycemia (see Insulin and Diabetes Pills section) and your blood glucose is below 90mg/dl, you should ingest 15–30 grams of carbohydrates. Speak with your health care provider to reduce the dose of your diabetes pills on days of exercise to prevent hypoglycemia and promote weight loss.[7]
- If you are on multiple daily injections, reduce the rapid acting insulin dose by 30–50 percent at the meal close to the exercise/physical activity time to avoid hypoglycemia.[9]
- If you are on an insulin pump, reduce your basal rate by 30–50 percent thirty to sixty minutes before exercise/physical activity in order to start exercising at blood glucose of 110mg/dl or above. Also, reduce your bolus by one to two units at the meal close to the exercise session/physical activity. The adjustments of both basal and bolus will be based on your own personal experience and blood glucose patterns.[39]
- If you have Type 1 diabetes and your blood glucose before exercise is 250mg/dl or above, check for ketones. You can use urine sticks that can be purchased in the pharmacy or a meter that requires a specific strip to check for ketones by a simple blood test. If the presence of ketones is positive, do not exercise and follow "sick day" rules as given to you by your health care provider. If the presence of ketones is negative and you feel well, you can exercise, however, check blood glucose and ketones half way through the activity and at the end of activity.[39]
- If your blood glucose level increases above the starting point value, be careful when taking a correction dose. If your blood glucose stays high for several hours you may take a reduced correction dose to avoid hypoglycemia several hours after exercise/physical activity.
- If you have Type 2 diabetes, you are not feeling well, you do not use insulin, and your blood glucose is close to or above 400mg/dl, you should not exercise.
- If you have Type 2 diabetes and you use insulin, follow the guidelines for insulin adjustments as listed above for Type 1 diabetes, however, you do not need to check for ketones. However, if you take insulin and diabetes pills, you should follow a blood glucose target of 110mg/dl or above before and after exercise/physical activity.

2. Carry snacks that contain 15–30 grams of carbohydrates, such as fruit, juice, or glucose tablets for the treatment of hypoglycemia.[7] Ice cream, cookies, chocolate, or any food that contain fat is not recommended for the treatment of hypoglycemia.
3. Drink fluids before, during, and after activity, and throughout the day. Dehydration affects blood glucose, therefore fluids are essential during exercise. You should always have a water bottle with you.

4. Avoid exercise in extreme heat. Wear loose and light clothing. If you experience signs of overheating, such as palpitations, cramps, headache, dizziness, nausea, or fainting, you must stop exercising.[13]

5. Avoid exercise in cold weather. If you choose to exercise outside, wear several layers to stay warm, gloves, and a hat. Wear shoes that provide good traction to prevent slips and pay attention to the walking surface to prevent falls.

6. Carry medical identification.[7]

7. When you exercise, wear polyester or blend (cotton-polyester) socks and use silica gel or air mid-soles and select shoes that fit well to your feet.

8. Do not push yourself to exercise at a higher intensity than you are comfortable with. If you experience joint or muscle pain, or chest discomfort, you should stop exercising and call your health care provider. Just listen to your body.[13]

9. If you are sick, take time off to heal, and resume activity at a much lower intensity, and progress slowly to higher intensity.[13]

FUTURE CONSIDERATIONS

Exercise and physical activity are major components in the prevention and management of diabetes and provides you with many benefits that will improve your overall health. Exercise can also help you to reduce the amount of medications you need to take as you become more active.

Aerobic, resistance, and stretching are the three important types of exercises that should be included in your exercise plan. Each one of these will provide you with different benefits that will help achieve your goals: prevent diabetes, manage diabetes, lose weight, feel better, and improve quality of life. If you plan ahead and reduce the insulin dosage on days you exercise/are physically active, this will help prevent hypoglycemia. By avoiding hypoglycemia, you will not need to eat or drink additional calories that especially beneficial if you are trying to lose weight.

When starting an exercise plan, consider the following:

1. Speak with your doctor to get clearance before starting an exercise plan.
2. Identify your barriers and find solutions.
3. Choose activities that are safe and enjoyable for you.
4. Set small, realistic goals so you will be able to achieve them.
5. Get support from your family and friends
6. Keep records of your blood glucose, the exercise program, and what you eat. Report to your health care provider/CDE in order to adjust your insulin/ diabetes pill dosage as you become more active.

As you follow these instructions and carefully progress with your exercise plan, you will see results and achieve your long-term goals. You just need to take the first step.

REFERENCES

1. Sanders LJ. "From Thebes to Toronto and the 21st century: An incredible journey." *Diabetes Spectrum* 15 (2002): 56–60.

2. MacCracken J, Hoel D. "From ants to analogues: Puzzles and promises in diabetes management." *Postgraduate Medicine* 101 (1997): 138–140, 143–145, 149–150.

3. Albright A, Franz M, Hornsby G, Kriska A, Marrero D, Ullrich I, Verity LS. "American College of Sports Medicine Position Stand. Exercise and Type 2 diabetes." *Medicine and Science in Sports Exercise* 32(7) (July 2000):1345–1360.

4. Morrato EH, Hill JO, Wyatt HR, Ghushchyan V, Sullivan PW. "Physical activity in U.S. adults with diabetes and at risk for developing diabetes, 2003." *Diabetes Care* 30 (2007): 203–209.

5. Gillies CL, Abrams KR, Lambert PC, Cooper NJ, Sutton AJ, Hsu RT, Khunti K. "Pharmacological and lifestyle interventions to prevent or delay Type 2 diabetes in people with impaired glucose tolerance: Systematic review and meta-analysis." *BMJ* 334 (2007): 299.

6. Kim SH, Lee SJ, Kang ES, Kang S, Hur KY, Lee HJ, Ahn CW, Cha BS, Yoo JS, Lee HC. "Effects of lifestyle modification on metabolic parameters and carotid intima-media thickness in patients with Type 2 diabetes mellitus." *Metabolism* 55 (2006): 1053–1059.

7. Mullooly CA, Chalmers KH. "Diabetes management therapies: Physical activity/exercise." In *A CORE Curriculum for Diabetes Education: Diabetes and Complications*, 5th edition. Franz MJ, ed. (Chicago: American Association of Diabetes Educators, 2003), pp. 61–90.

8. Hamdy O, Goodyear L, Horton ES. "Diet and exercise in Type 2 diabetes." *Endocrinology and Metabolism Clinics of North America* 30 (2001): 883–907.

9. Steppel JH, Horton WS. "Exercise in patients with Diabetes Mellitus." *Joslin's Diabetes Mellitus*, 14th ed. (Philadelphia, PA: Lippincott Williams & Wilkins, 2005).

10. Beaser RS. *Joslin's Diabetes Deskbook. A Guide for Primary Care Providers* (Boston, MA Joslin Diabetes Center, 2003).

11. American Diabetes Association (2007). "Standards of medical care in diabetes. Clinical Practice Recommendations 2007." *Diabetes Care* 30(Supplement 1): S4–S41.

12. U.S. Department of Health and Human Services. Centers for Disease Control and Prevention, Division of Nutrition and Physical Activity. *Promoting Physical Activity: A Guide for Community Action* (Champaign, IL, Human Kinetics, 1999).

13. Frontera W, Bean J (Eds.). Strength and Power Training: *A Guide for Adults of All Ages.* (Boston, MA: Harvard Health Publications, 2005).

14. Dunstan DW, Daly RM, Owen N, Jolley D, De Courten M, Shaw J, Zimmet P. "High-intensity resistance training improves glycemic control in older patients with Type 2 diabetes." *Diabetes Care* 25 (2002): 1729–1736.

15. Dunstan DW, Vulikh E, Owen N, Jolley D, Shaw J, Zimmet P. "Community center-based resistance training for the maintenance of glycemic control in adults with Type 2 diabetes." *Diabetes Care* 29 (2006): 2586–2591.

16. Gaesser GA. "Exercise for prevention and treatment of cardiovascular disease, Type 2 diabetes, and metabolic syndrome." *Current Diabetes Report* 7 (2007): 14–19.

17. Shen W, Punyanitya M, Chen J, Gallagher D, Albua J, Pi-Sunyer X, Lewis CE, Grunfeld C, Heshka S, Heymsfield S. "Waist circumference correlates with metabolic syndrome indicators better than percentage fat." *Obesity* 14 (2006): 727–736.

18. Torpy J. "The metabolic syndrome." *The Journal of the American Medical Association* 295 (2006): 850.

19. "Diabetes Surveillance Report, 1999". Centers for Disease Control and Prevention, U.S. Department of Health and Human Services.

20. Fritz T, Wandell P, Aberg H, and Engfeldt P. "Walking for exercise—does three times per week influence risk factors in Type 2 diabetes?" *Diabetes Res Clin Pract* 71 (2006): 21–27.

21. American College of Sports Medicine. *ACSM's Guidelines for Exercise Testing and Prescription*, 7th ed. (Baltimore, MD: Lippincott Williams and Wilkins, 2006).

22. Lee S, Kuk JL, Katzmarzyk PT, Blair SN, Church TS, Ross R. "Cardiorespiratory fitness attenuates metabolic risk independent of abdominal subcutaneous and visceral fat in men." *Diabetes Care* 28 (2005): 895–901.

23. Balducci S, Iacobellis G, Parisi L, Di Biase N, Calandriello E, Leonetti F, Fallucca F. "Exercise training can modify the natural history of diabetic peripheral neuropathy." *J Diabetes Complications* 20 (2006): 216–223.

24. Loreto CD, Fanelli C, Murdolo G, De Cicco A, Parlanti N, Ranchelli A, Fatone C, Taglioni C, Santeusanio F, De Feo P. "Make your diabetic patients walk." *Diabetes Care* 28(6) (June 2005): 1295–1302.

25. Hu G, Jousilahti P, Barengo NC, Qiao Q, Lakka TA, Tuomilehto J. "Physical activity, cardiovascular risk factors, and mortality among Finnish adults with diabetes." *Diabetes Care* 28 (2005): 799–805.

26. Howley ET, Franks BD. *Health Fitness Instructor's Handbook*, 3rd ed. (Champaign, IL: Human Kinetics, 1997).

27. Brubaker PH, Kaminsky LA, Whaley MH. *Coronary Artery Disease: Essentials of Prevention and Rehabilitation Programs* (Champaign, IL: Human Kinetics, 2002).

28. Vinik AI, Tomris E. "Recognizing and treating diabetic autonomic neuropathy." *Cleveland Clinic Journal of Medicine* 68 (2001): 928–944.

29. Gonder LA, Zrebiec J. "Diabetes management therapies: Hypoglycemia." In *A CORE Curriculum for Diabetes Education: Diabetes and Complications*, 5th edition. Franz MJ, ed. (Chicago, IL: American Association of Diabetes Educators, 2003), pp. 279–310.

30. Haskell WL, Lee I, Pate RR, Powell KE, Blair SN, Franklin BA, Macera CA, Heath GW, Thompson PD. "Physical activity and public health: Updated recommendations for adults from the American College of Sports Medicine and American Heart Association." *Circulation* 116 (2007): 1081–1093.

31. Baechle TR, Earle RW. *Essentials of Strength Training and Conditioning*, 2nd ed. (Champaign, IL: Human Kinetics, 2002).

32. Levine SD, Rice D, Pagels M, et al. "effect of interval training on hemoglobin A1c levels in obese adults with Type II diabetes." *Medicine & Science in Sports & Exercise* 29(Supplement) (1997): 92.

33. Tjonna AE et al. "Superior cardiovascular effect of interval training versus moderate exercise in patients with metabolic syndrome." *Medicine and Science in Sports and Exercise* 39 (2007): S173.

34. Eves ND, Plotnikoff RC. "Resistance training and Type 2 diabetes: Considerations for implementation at the population level." *Diabetes Care* 29 (2006): 1933–1941.

35. Sahay BK. "Role of yoga in diabetes." *J Assoc Physicians India* 55 (2007): 121–126.

36. Persinger R, Foster C, Gibson M, et al. "Consistency of the Talk Test for exercise prescription." *Medicine & Science in Sports & Exercise* 36 (2004): 1632–1636.

37. Division of Nutrition and Physical Activity, National Center for Chronic Disease Prevention and Health Promotion, August 26, 2006.

38. Mullooly C and the staff of the Joslin Diabetes Center. *Staying Healthy with Diabetes: Physical Activity & Fitness* (Boston, MA: Joslin Diabetes Center, 2006).

39. Steppel JH, Horton WS. "Exercise for the patient with Type 1 Diabetes Mellitus." *Diabetes Mellitus: A Fundamental and Clinical Text*, 3rd ed. (Philadelphia, PA: Lippincott Williams & Wilkins, 2004).

40. Shaw J. "The deadliest sin." *Harvard Magazine.* March–April, 2004.

10

EXERCISE AND ARTHRITIS

Philip Blount

BACKGROUND

Rheumatological diseases affect nearly 43 million Americans. That is about one in every six people. Physicians recognize rheumatologic conditions as being one of the most prevalent chronic disabling conditions affecting our population. During the past ten to fifteen years, new treatments have been developed in managing arthritis. These include the use of disease-modifying antirheumatic drugs, recommending exercise instead of relative rest, and an increased practice of rehabilitation principles early in the disease course. Doctors are discovering that exercise has a vital role in the management of patients with rheumatologic conditions. Exercise is now considered an effective intervention in rheumatologic conditions and is an important component of primary prevention. This chapter will examine the current exercise studies on arthritis and present a rehabilitation approach to the rheumatic patient focusing on how exercise can be incorporated into a comprehensive management plan.[1]

Of course it is well known that exercise carries significant health benefits, such as decreasing the risks of several chronic diseases, increasing longevity, improving psychological health, and enhancing quality of life.[3] Exercise is so beneficial, even people with arthritis should regularly participate. But what is exercise? When we begin to talk about exercise, it is important to define our terms. Exercise, for the purpose of this chapter, will be defined as *a bodily exertion for the sake of a specific adaptive response.* There are several specific adaptive responses that are enhanced with exercise training such as aerobic capacity, muscular strength, muscular endurance, flexibility, and balance. All of these adaptive responses are measurable and progress can be recorded in a training diary as follows:

1. Flexibility—Measure and record range-of-motion of each joint.
2. Strength—Record the resistance (weight), number of repetitions, or time engaged in each set (using a stopwatch).
3. Aerobic capacity—Record the amount of time (minutes) activity is sustained.

With the wide variety of exercise activities available, it is important to remember there is no one universal program to meet all of these needs. Specific goals should therefore be established. For an exercise program to be successful for an individual, there should be a measurable improvement in the individual's goal response. Physical activity that does not result in a measurable improvement or that is done strictly for fun could be classified as a recreational activity and not exercise according to this definition.

A typical exercise session consists of a warm-up, a training period, and a cool-down.[3] A warm-up serves to prepare the body for exercise. In general, the warm-up serves to increase core body temperature making the muscles and soft tissues more pliable. The warm-up also prepares the circulatory and nervous systems for exercise. This is followed by the training session, which can emphasize flexibility, strengthening, and aerobic training. A cool-down is then performed to return the body back to homeostasis and heart rate back to a normal level. All three phases can be individualized based on the practitioner's exercise goals, time constraints, and interests.

Flexibility Training: "Time to Limber Up!"

When muscles are shorter than their ideal length, they are at a biomechanical disadvantage when they are required to generate force.[3] Flexibility training is a form of exercise designed to increase range of motion and lengthen shortened muscles and tendons. Flexibility training involves various type of stretching activities that can be performed alone, with equipment, or with a partner. Flexibility training has been shown not only to possibly prevent injury but can also result in a relative strength increase by placing muscles at an optimal biomechanical advantage. Targeted joints should be moved through their full available range of motion at least once per day however, it has been suggested that flexibility exercises should be performed as many as three to five times per day. Increasing range of motion requires stretching the targeted muscle through its full range of pain free motion and holding for at least thirty seconds. Stretching exercises are typically performed after a warming-up, which optimizes the elastic qualities of the musculotendinous region. This can be performed actively by first performing some gentle exercises to increase body temperature or artificially by applying superficial heat to the affected area.

Strength Training: "Stronger Muscles Mean Safer Joints!"

Strength development through resistance training is important for maintaining functional capacity, preventing and recovering from injury, and even improving sports performance. A muscle can lose 30 percent of its bulk in a week and up to 5 percent of its strength per day when maintained on strict bed rest.[4] The medical literature provides ample evidence that muscles can be strengthened, even in patients with rheumatic diseases.[5] Strengthening of a muscle can be achieved in several ways. The most well-known type of strengthening program consists of isotonic muscular contractions. An isotonic muscle contraction is dynamic in which the limbs and joints move through a range of motion. There is a lifting phase and a lowering phase. These types of contractions are seen with strength training involving free weights, elastic bands, or machines. The typical isotonic strengthening program includes exercises where a body part is moving through a full range of motion with enough resistance to cause fatigue in the targeted muscle within eight to twelve repetitions. One to three sets of the exercise are performed.[6]

Not so well known is isometric strength training. An isometric contraction is one in which the muscle length does not change and the limbs do not move; only muscle tension is generated. An example of an isometric exercise would be pushing your foot into the ground while seated, flexing and tensing the thigh muscles, or pressing your palms together tensing the pectoral muscles. Isometric exercises are ideally suited for restoring and maintaining strength in patients with arthritic joints. A recommended isometric program involves three daily maximal contractions, each held for approximately six seconds with twenty seconds of rest between each.[7] Isometric strengthening programs have shown to increase quadriceps strength in patients with rheumatoid arthritis up to 27 percent.[8] Strengthening the muscles through isometric or isotonic exercise will help protect the joints in the arthritic patient by supporting the joint and the surrounding ligamentous structures.

Aerobic Training: "Put an End to Fatigue!"

Simply stated, the global effect of an aerobic training response is to increase the capacity of the heart and skeletal muscles to perform work. Improving this capacity can lead to an increased functional level in patients suffering from arthritic conditions.[9] Aerobic exercise has been proven to be safe and beneficial in patients with rheumatic diseases.[10] The primary focus should be on adopting an activity and progression that will result in long-term participation. Most studies suggest that a person can experience a 15 percent or greater improvement in aerobic capacity within three months of regular aerobic training.[2] Optimal exercises for the arthritic patient are low-impact and include walking, cycling, or swimming that incorporate a large muscle mass. The recommended exercise intensity range is from 55 percent to 80 percent of the maximum heart rate. This can easily be estimated by taking (220 − your age in years) × 0.55 or 0.80. This typically translates to a rating of perceived exertion between "fairly light" and "hard." Aerobic training typically includes three to five sessions per week of twenty minutes or more of continuous activity. The intensity, duration, and frequency of the aerobic exercise prescription can be modified based on the patient's goals and also to enhance compliance.[2]

"Variety and Individualization Is the Key!"

It is important to realize that there is no one universal exercise program to maximize benefits in all areas. For example, a progressive stationary cycling program will result in an aerobic training response and increase lower limb strength and endurance but may not improve flexibility or upper body strength or endurance. Additionally, it is also possible to achieve a desired outcome through multiple training strategies. For example, strengthening of the muscles can occur from using body-weight or household objects for resistance, elastic bands, or variable resistance exercise machines at a health club. This opens the door to exploring the vast array of exercise activities in order to individualize a program for each specific person. Before incorporating an exercise program, it is important to have specific goals. All exercise follows a "specific adaptation to imposed demand," or SAID principle.[11] The most effective exercise program is one that most closely resembles the desired functional task one wishes to improve.

One obvious problem with exercise prescription is that of compliance. Several common barriers to exercise compliance exist, such as the time commitment involved, a lack of interest, or fear of injury, or self-consciousness.[2] Compliance can be optimized by clearly outlining the specific benefits of the exercise program in relation to the patient's specific diagnosis. Typically, the exercise prescription is individualized according to personal preference, goals, and daily lifestyle of the patient to enhance compliance.

ARTHRITIS AND EXERCISE

Simply stated, arthritis is defined as a disorder of the joints. The term "arthritis" comes from the Greek *arthron* meaning joints and "*itis*" meaning inflammation. Today's physicians normally classify arthritis into two broad categories, noninflammatory and inflammatory arthritis. It is crucial that the patient knows what type of arthritis has been diagnosed before beginning an exercise program. In order to do this, a physician may perform a history and physical examination, order blood work, urinalysis, x-rays, and even joint fluid analysis. The primary goals in the rehabilitation of patients with arthritic conditions are to educate patients on their disease process, understand joint preservation techniques to decrease pain, improve flexibility and range of motion, and increase muscular strength and endurance.[12]

OSTEOARTHRITIS (OA)

Osteoarthritis, or OA, is the most common noninflammatory arthritis. It is also the most common form of arthritis. Osteoarthritis is sometimes called "degenerative joint disease" and results from wear and tear on the joints much like the tread of an old tire. Typically, OA affects the weight bearing joints such as the knee, hip, and the spine. The majority of adults over the age of 55 have some form of OA. The cause of OA is uncertain but there are known risk factors that lead to the development of OA such as prior joint injury, malalignment, obesity, and weak supporting muscles. A typical presentation of a patient with osteoarthritis includes joint pain, limited range of motion, and occasional swelling. The only known cure for osteoarthritis is joint replacement surgery. However, with proper education, medications, and exercise, osteoarthritis can be successfully managed. Exercise can not only assist in pain reduction, but also maximize function, improve strength and endurance, and provide a sense of well-being.[3]

The primary goals in osteoarthritis management include patient education of the disease process, improving flexibility, and increasing muscular strength and endurance. A range of motion assessment and flexibility should be the first step in exercise prescription for the patient with osteoarthritis. To assess the range of motion of the various joints the following simple tests can be performed:

- *Shoulder:* To measure shoulder rotation, try the complex motion of reaching behind your back and trying to scratch an itch, sometimes called the *Apley Scratch Test.* This functional motion is required in daily activities such as reaching into a back pocket, bathing, or fastening clothes. Typically, people are able to come within a few inches of the opposite shoulder blade. The dominant arm typically reaches less than the nondominant.
- *Lower Back:* To test the extension of the lumbar spine, lean backwards as far as possible. The amount of extension is measured from the trunk line and vertical line. Normally, 20–30 degrees of extension is possible without pain. Loss of low back range of motion might be an early indicator of developing osteoarthritis.
- *Knees:* Lying on your back, flex the knees as far as possible. Normally, you should be able to bring your knee close to your buttock or even touch it. This corresponds to an angle of approximately 130–150 degrees. Flexion to 110 degrees is usually sufficient to allow individuals to climb or descend stairs and to complete other activities of daily living. Comparing the heel to buttock distance on both sides is a good way to assess the loss of flexion. Often, loss of flexion is due to joint swelling or arthritic changes within the knee.
- *Hips:* Early degenerative changes in the hips may be detected through an assessment of hip rotation. Hip rotation is where an extended leg is turned in and out. People with early degenerative arthritis of the hip joints frequently lose rotation in the affected hip before losing flexion or abduction. They may also experience groin pain that limits passive rotation.

Flexibility limitations in the lower limbs contribute to mobility deficiencies such as walking. Flexibility limitations in the upper limbs can affect activities of daily living such as dressing. It is important to realize that a limited range of motion in one joint can be associated with problems in other joints along the kinetic chain. A clear example is osteoarthritis of the knee. Limited knee range of motion results in adaptive changes in both the hip and the ankle, thereby reducing the overall efficiency and kinematics during gait. The affected joints should be moved through their available range of motion and statically stretched for thirty seconds at least three times per day. In the case of knee arthritis, specific stretches for the hip flexors, hamstrings, and calves should be used.[1]

Approximately twenty years ago, prescriptions for rehabilitation avoided any activities that would increase joint loading. It is now clear that joint movement and loading are essential for proper stimulation of the joint. Research focusing on resistance exercises has shown that patients with osteoarthritis who perform strength training have dramatic improvement in muscle strength, endurance, and contractions of the muscles surrounding the arthritic joint.[13] In the case of lower limb osteoarthritis, such as the hip or the knee, strength training should focus on isotonic closed kinetic chain exercise. A closed kinetic chain exercise for the lower limb is where the foot remains stationary while movement occurs at the ankle, knee, and hip joint. Examples of such exercise include the leg press or the squat. These movements involve multiple muscle groups and replicate activities of daily living, such as getting up from a chair or climbing stairs. Leg presses effectively strengthen the quadriceps muscles and are thus beneficial to patient suffering from knee osteoarthritis. The following general rules can be used as a guide to perform leg presses. However, the physician or therapist should be consulted for the best exercise for one's specific condition.

1. The leg press is better than the free-squat for those with patellofemoral arthritis or those with anterior knee pain.
2. When leg pressing, a wide stance is better than a narrow stance for those with anterior knee pain.
3. Working from a 0 to 60 degree angle when performing leg presses is generally well tolerated for those with anterior knee pain. Working up to 100 degrees of knee flexion can be performed, but it is not recommended for the thighs to go beyond parallel during the movement. In other words, do not perform deep leg presses.

Closed kinetic chain strengthening exercises for the thigh have been examined under laboratory conditions. An article published in *Medicine Science and Sports and Exercise* in 2001 looked at knee biomechanics during the squatting exercise. Patellofemoral compressive forces and tibiofemoral compressive forces increase as knees flex and decrease as knees are extended, reaching a peak value near maximum knee flexion. Based on this study, recommendations for training in the squat are to exercise between 0 and 50 degrees in order to minimize forces across the knee joint. The author concluded that the squat was shown to be an effective exercise to utilize during knee arthritis rehabilitation.[14]

Patients with osteoarthritis can also benefit from aerobic exercises, as long as their symptoms are not exacerbated. Patients with lower limb osteoarthritis, such as the knee, are often unable to tolerate high volumes of aerobic activity. An alternative method would be to include several short sessions per day. The American College of Sports Medicine recommends beginning with ten minutes per day of continuous activity. A systematic increase (two to five minutes per week) will allow time for the adaptive changes to occur and minimize overuse-type pain. A goal of thirty continuous minutes of aerobic exercise is optimal. Studies have shown that an aerobic training effect can be seen with such an approach.[15]

Case #1: Noninflammatory Arthritis

Robert is a 62-year-old, right-hand-dominant contractor who has a chief complaint of pain in both of his knees. His pain is located in the front of the knee, but also in the joint. He describes his symptoms as "stiff first thing in the morning" and "aching after a long day." He is often required by his job to kneel and squat, which exacerbates his symptoms, but even weather changes have been known to make his knees hurt. Robert sustained a football injury during college, which required an arthroscopic surgical procedure on the right knee with partial meniscectomy. Robert has found relief with rest, using over-the-counter antiinflammatories, and occasional over-the-counter glucosamine and chondroitin sulfate. Robert currently weighs 235 pounds at 5 foot 10 inches. He has pain daily but is mostly concerned about a trip next summer to Disney World with his three grandchildren.

Robert's physiatrist performed a detailed history and thorough physical exam. It is noted on simple inspection that Robert's knees show mild swelling and malalignment. Range of motion testing reveals the inability to fully extend the right knee, but knee flexion is fully preserved. Robert walked up and down the hall and performed some simple examination tests in the office to evaluate for bilateral hip flexor and Achilles tendon tightness. X-rays revealed joint space narrowing, in the medial compartment and the formation of osteophytes or bone spurs. Robert's physiatrist diagnosed him with bilateral knee osteoarthritis.

A dialog occurred between Robert and the physiatrist to discuss nonoperative management options. For his pain control, Robert's physiatrist outlined the use of simple medications, prescribed physical therapy to instruct him on the use of modalities, and evaluated him for orthotics to help with alignment. Next, Robert's physiatrist referred him to a registered dietician with a goal of a 10 percent weight loss over the next six to eight months. Further discussion regarding injection therapy is discussed. For exercise the physiatrist's specific goals include increasing Robert's quadriceps strength to offer joint protection, maintaining a desired weight, and improving flexibility throughout the entire kinetic chain. Robert is most concerned about his vacation and his specific goal is to decrease his pain while improving his endurance for the walking involved at Disney World. When exercise is discussed, Robert admits to two common errors to compliance. He complains of time constraints and the lack of access as he is not a member of a health club facility. Robert's exercise prescription is therefore individualized, taking his goals and needs into account.

Robert's exercise prescription consists of a warm-up, a training session, and a cool-down period. Due to Robert's lack of access to a fitness facility, his therapist recommends the purchase of a $25 Physio-Ball. Robert's warm-up can be performed using the Physio-Ball to increase his core temperature, stretch his hip flexors and hamstrings, strengthen his abdominals and low back, and provide a general warm-up prior to his training session. His therapist is able to review these warm-up exercises with him and supply him with both written instructions and detailed pictures. He is instructed to use this warm-up before each training session. His training phase will have two components. The first will be a strengthening program. Robert's physical therapist recommends closed kinetic chain quadriceps exercises where the feet remain stable while motion occurs at the hip and knee joint. First, Robert is taught an exercise called "Wall Squats" where he leans against the wall and supports his body weight using his thigh muscles. No movement is occurring at the hip and knee and, therefore, this is termed an isometric closed kinetic chain exercise. As Robert is able, he progresses the intensity of this simple exercise by increasing the amount of time each "Wall Squat" is sustained. He is also taught to increase the angle of his knee joint by squatting lower as pain allows. With time being so valuable to Robert, he is instructed how to incorporate this exercise into numerous daily activities such as while brushing his teeth or returning phone calls. An isotonic closed kinetic chain exercise for the quadriceps can be performed using the Physio-Ball. Robert places the Physio-Ball between his back and the wall and he completes dynamic Wall Squats, three to five sets of fifteen repetitions each. With movement occurring at the hip and knee joints, this becomes an isotonic closed kinetic chain exercise. Progression can be made with the number of repetitions, number of sets, added resistance, and can even be progressed to an advanced single leg wall squat. Robert has been instructed to perform quadriceps strengthening exercises two to three times per week and his therapist reminds him that this program should take no longer than ten to fifteen minutes.

Since Robert will primarily be walking at Disney World, his aerobic training will be specific to that goal. A walking program is designed instead of stationary cycling, elliptical trainer, or treadmill walking. Robert is currently unable to tolerate walks longer than twenty to thirty minutes secondary to his knee pain, so his prescription will be modified. Robert will perform several short walks per day, which is easily tolerated, instead of a single long session. This will prevent Robert's knees from aching from one prolonged activity but will provide a training response if his overall volume is progressed. At home, Robert begins with a short walk before breakfast and another after dinner. At work, Robert is able to park far away from his office and has found time during the day to take one walking break. The goal of each session is to perform ten to fifteen minutes of walking gradually increasing his overall daily volume. Comfortable walking shoes are recommended for joint protection, and his goal is to be able to perform several ten to fifteen minute walks per day, three to five days per week. He is advised to perform his aerobic training program on opposite days of his strengthening.

Robert's cool-down phase will have two components, both intrinsic and extrinsic cool-down. After the end of a training session, Robert is instructed to perform static stretches for his hip flexors, quadriceps, hamstrings, and Achilles tendons. He holds each stretch for approximately thirty seconds without bouncing. This serves to lower his heart rate. His extrinsic cool-down following training involves ice. Icing the knees after exercise not only cools the affected joint, but also helps reduce swelling and relieve pain.

Robert is asked by his health care providers to keep a training log and to comment on any symptom exacerbations. He is also asked about his exercise on return visits. It is over halfway to the Disney World vacation and Robert has lost weight and his exercise tolerance has improved greatly. He feels very confident that he will be able to participate fully and enjoy the family vacation.

INFLAMMATORY ARTHRITIS

Rheumatoid arthritis or RA is the most common inflammatory arthritis. Although the exact cause is unknown, it is thought that RA is a condition where the body attacks itself by mistake. RA is more common in women, age 30–50, and not only affects the hands, wrists, elbows and shoulders, but other organ systems as well. Fatigue is one of the most common complaints in RA. RA is not to be confused with OA. RA is managed differently by rheumatologists and early aggressive treatment is now the standard of care. Critical to the management of RA should be an exercise program aimed at preventing disability and preserving or improving function.[16]

Common complaints in patients with RA include fatigue, pain, decreased aerobic capacity, decreased strength, and decreased range of motion.[16] The primary goals in the rehabilitation of patients with RA are to educate the patient on the disease process, teach energy conservation techniques, and recommend exercises focusing on improving flexibility, and maximizing range of motion of the affected joints.

A therapist can provide instruction on an appropriate warm-up followed by gentle stretching exercises. Low to moderate intensity aerobic training should also be encouraged. Studies have shown that low to moderate intensity aerobic exercise can improve aerobic capacity, thus decreasing fatigue in patients with RA without increasing inflammation.[16] A common mode of exercise for this purpose is pool therapy. The buoyancy of the water supports the body weight and decreases the stress across the joints in the lower extremities. Exercising in warm water also provides local and systemic relaxation and decreases pain.[16] Pool therapy is now becoming a popular mode for exercise in patients with inflammatory arthritis. Strengthening can also be accomplished with isometric and isotonic type exercises. Isometric exercises are typically tried first. Patients are instructed to tense the muscles without moving the joints several times per day. When progressing to isotonic exercises intensity (the amount of resistance and number of sets) should be kept very low, as dynamic high intensity isotonic exercise has the potential for exacerbating inflammation.[16] Isotonic strengthening exercises should not be performed during an inflammatory exacerbation. Joints should be rested during acute flares.[16] A brace or orthotic can be used to help rest a joint. Modalities such as superficial heating or icing used as part of an extrinsic warm-up or cool-down can also assist in pain control. Rheumatoid arthritis is a chronic disease that needs continued physical exercise to prevent muscle and functional deterioration.

Case #2: Inflammatory Arthritis

Karen is a 34-year-old, right-hand-dominant office administrator. Her chief complaint is that of fatigue, morning stiffness, and wrist and hand pain. All of her symptoms are worse with activity such as gardening, but now her symptoms are interfering with her work. She denies any symptoms such as chills, rash or gastrointestinal complaint, but has admitted to a low grade temperature in the past. Her primary care provider has referred her to a rheumatologist, who has diagnosed rheumatoid arthritis and started her on medications. She presents to her physiatrist with a goal of improving her functional capacity to where she can make it through the day with more stamina.

Her physiatrist reviewed her medical record, family history, and current medications in order to identify any contraindications to exercise. Then, a thorough physical exam with emphasis on joint range of motion was performed. A dialog occurred between the physiatrist and the patient regarding the patient's goals and the patient's management strategy. The physiatrist's specific goals are to maintain range of motion, improve aerobic capacity, and educate Karen on the disease process, including symptom exacerbation. A thorough evaluation of the hand and wrist joints was performed and a referral to a hand therapist was made for education on superficial heating and icing, range of motion stretching exercises, establishment of a home exercise program, and evaluation for custom splints for joint protection. Compliance issues to exercise are also discussed and it is discovered that Karen does have access to a health club facility with pool.

Karen is prescribed pool therapy two days per week. This is done in a group setting with an instructor supervising. She is able to incorporate this into her weekly routine. The group dynamic provides accountability and not only has she made new friends, but she has also learned from others practical tips on management of her arthritis. Karen performs isometric strengthening exercises for her limbs and core strengthening exercises taught to her by her therapist. These can be performed at home or at work because they require no special equipment. She can effectively rest her joints with custom hand splints. By wearing these at night, she is literally treating her joints in her sleep. Most importantly, Karen is now applying energy conservation techniques (see the subsection on the techniques to prevent arthritis pain) into her lifestyle, which helps with her fatigue. Karen would admit she is not an athlete, but her individualized exercise program has enhanced her quality of life by giving her more endurance and strength. She feels empowered in her new management knowledge of her arthritic condition. Listed below are seven techniques to prevent arthritis pain[17] (courtesy of MayoClinic.com).

1. Move each joint through its full pain free range of motion at least once a day.
   This will help you maintain range of motion in your joints. The amount you are able to move each joint without pain may vary from day to day. Therefore, take care not to overdo it. Keep movement slow and gentle. Sudden jerking or bouncing may hurt your joints.
2. Learn to understand and respect your arthritis pain.
   Understand the difference between general discomfort of arthritis and pain from overusing the joint. By noting the activities that stress the joint, you can avoid repeating that movement. Arthritis pain that lasts more than an hour after an activity may indicate that the activity was too stressful. Remember that you are more likely to damage your joints when they are painful and swollen.
3. Be careful how you use your hands.
   You use your fingers in many day-to-day activities. Stressful positions and activities may increase the risk of developing hand deformities. You can perform most tasks in easier ways that put less stress forces on your joints.
   (a) Avoid positions that push your other fingers toward your little finger. Finger motion should be in the direction of your thumb whenever possible. For example, don't brush crumbs off the table with your palm flat on the table. Instead, turn your hand so that the little finger is resting on the table and palm is facing you that push the crumbs off the table.
   (b) Avoid making a tight fist. Use sticks or built up handles on tools, which make them easier to hold.
   (c) Avoid pinching items between your thumb and your fingers. Hold a book, plate, or mug in the palms of your hand. If you are reading for long periods, use a book holder. Instead of a handheld purse, use one with a shoulder strap.
4. Use good body mechanics.
   The way you carry your body largely affects how much strain you put on your joints. Proper body mechanics allows you to use your body more efficiently and conserve energy.
   (a) When you are sitting, the proper height for a work surface is two inches below your bent elbow. Make sure you have good back and foot support when you sit. Your forearms and upper legs should be level with the floor.
   (b) If you type at a keyboard for long periods and your chair doesn't have arms, consider using wrist or forearm supports. An angled work surface for reading and writing is easy on your neck.
   (c) When you are standing, the height of your work surface should enable you to work comfortably without stooping.
   (d) Increase the height of your chair to decrease stress on your hips and knees as you get up and down.

(e) To pick up items off the floor, stoop by using the knees and hips or sit on a chair and bend over.

(f) Carry heavy objects close to your chest, supporting the weight on your forearms.

(g) Maintain good posture. Posture causes uneven weight distribution and may strain ligaments and muscles.

5. Use the strongest joint available for the job.

Save your weaker joints for the specific job that only they can accomplish. Throughout the day, favor your large joints. For example, carry objects with your palms open, distributing the weight equally over your forearms. Slide objects along the counter or work bench, rather than lifting them. When opening cabinets, use a loop that you can pull with your wrist or forearm to decrease stress on your fingers.

6. Avoid keeping your joints in the same position for prolonged periods of time.

Don't give your joints a chance to become stiff. Keep them moving. When writing or doing hand work, release your grip every ten to fifteen minutes. On long car trips, get out of the car, stretch, and move around at least every hour. While watching television, get up and move around every half hour.

7. Balance periods of rest and activity during the day.

Effectively managing your workload throughout the day can help you avoid overworked joints. Work at a steady, moderate pace and avoid rushing. Rest before you become fatigued or sore. Alternate light and moderate activities throughout the day. Take a periodic stretch break.

If you have a diagnosis of arthritis and are not exercising, consider making an appointment with your physician to discuss the type of arthritis you have and ask about the many positive benefits regular exercise can provide. With guidance, an exercise prescription, such as the following, can be customized to meet your specific goals and to protect your joints.

1. Discuss with your health care provider your diagnosis, goals, and precautions before beginning an exercise program.
2. Incorporate both fitness and functional exercises in a comprehensive program.
3. During each exercise session, start with a brief warm-up then perform flexibility exercises for affected joints. Next, strength and endurance training, and finally aerobic activity.
4. Flexibility exercises can be performed one to two times daily, using the pain-free range of motion.
5. Perform strength training using one to three sets of twelve repetitions two to three days per week using pain threshold as an index of intensity.
6. With aerobic training, begin with short bouts (approximately ten minutes). Add five minutes per session up to a goal of thirty minutes. Low-impact activities, such as cycling, aquatic, and walking are preferred.
7. Avoid exercise during arthritic "flare-ups."
8. Stop exercise if you notice persistent fatigue, increased weakness, decreased range of motion, increased joint swelling, or discomfort that lasts longer than one hour after exercise.

Table 10.1
Summary of Exercise Programming[15]

Components	Frequency	Intensity	Duration	Activity
Flexibility	Minimal 2–3 d/wk Ideal 5–7 d/wk	Stretch to tightness at the end of the range of motion but not to pain	15–30 seconds	Static stretch all major muscle groups
Resistance	2–3 d/wk	Volitional fatigue OR stop 2–3 reps before volitional fatigue	1 set of 8–12	8–10 exercises include all major muscle groups
Cardiorespiratory	3–5 d/wk	50%/80% HR–max 12–16 RPE	20–60 min	Large muscle groups, dynamic activity

Source: American College of Sports Medicine. *Exercise Prescription & Testing*, 7th ed. (Baltimore, MD: Lippincott Williams & Wilkins, 2006).

Medications such as Tylenol (acetaminophen) and antiinflammatories are commonly prescribed for osteoarthritis. A physiatrist may assist in over-the-counter or prescription dosages. Glucosamine and chondroitin sulfate are vitamin supplements that can assist with the pain management in osteoarthritis. Glucosamine is a natural compound in your body that helps make your cartilage strong and rigid. Several different preparations are available over the counter at drug stores and health food stores. Osteoarthritis causes a breakdown of joint cartilage and can affect any joint. Because glucosamine is a component of normal cartilage, it is thought that glucosamine supplements may be able to help the body repair damaged cartilage. Glucosamine is worth a try for patients suffering from osteoarthritis. If no benefit is seen after a month or two of proper use, the supplement should be discontinued. If, however, benefit is noted, this may be a safe adjunct to a comprehensive osteoarthritis treatment plan.

No other arthritis treatment can boast the quality of life and functional improvements seen with an appropriate exercise prescription. Share with your health care professional your specific goals and interests. It is true that long-term exercise compliance is best when there is a clear understanding of the rationale and goals behind the exercise recommendations and when exercise can be incorporated into the individual's everyday life. Exercise can be safely tailored for flexibility to preserve and maximize range of motion, muscular strength to protect the joints, and aerobic capacity to help with overall endurance. Exercise principles of warm-up (superficial heat) and cool-down (icing) and relative rest (bracing) can be used both during training sessions and as a method of pain control. Learn how, when, and why to exercise with arthritis and empower yourself with physical medicine. Your body will thank you.

REFERENCES

1. Sisto SA, Malanga G. "Osteoarthritis and Therapeutic Exercise." *American Journal of Physical Medicine and Rehabilitation* 85 (2006):S69–S78.

2. American College of Sports Medicine. *Position Stand of Fitness: Healthy Adult.*

3. Stitik T. "Osteoarthritis." In *Physical Medicine & Rehabilitation: Principles and Practice,* 4th ed. DeLisa, J ed. (Philadelphia, PA: Lippincott Williams & Wilkins, 2005).

4. MacDougall JD, Elder GCB, Sale DG, Moroz JR, Sutton JR. "Effects of Strength Training and Immobilization on Human Muscle Fibers." *Eur J App Phys* 43 (1980):25–34.

5. Muller EA. "Influence of Training and Inactivity on Muscle Strength." *Arch Phys Med Rehabil* 51 (1970):440–462.

6. DeLoreme TL, Watkins AL. "Techniques of Progressive Resistance Exercise." *Arch Phys Med Rehabil* 29 (1948):263–273.

7. Liberson WT. "Brief Isometric Exercises in Therapeutic Exercise." *Therapeutic Exercise,* 4th ed. (Baltimore, MD: Williams and Wilkins, 1984).

8. Nordemar R. "Physical Training in Rheumatoid Arthritis. A Controlled Long Termed Study II." *Scand J Rheum* 10 (1981):25–30.

9. Clark HH. "Adaptations in Strength and Muscular Endurance Resulting from Exercise." In Wilmore JH (ed). *Exercise and Sport Sciences Reviews,* Vol. 1 (New York: Academic Press, 1973).

10. Nordemar R, Ekblom B, Zachrisson L, Lundgrist K. "Physical Training in Rheumatoid Arthritis. A Controlled Long Term Study I." *Scand J. Rheum* 10 (1981):17–23.

11. Atha J. "Strengthening Muscle." *Exercise and Sport Sciences Reviews,* Vol. 9 (Philadelphia, PA: The Franklin Inst. Press, 1981).

12. "Osteoarthritis Center," www.mayoclinic.com (accessed Dec. 29, 2007).

13. Beals CA, Lanyman RM, Banwell BF et al. "Measurement of Exercise Tolerance in Patients with Rheumatoid Arthritis and Osteoarthritis." *J Rheumatol* 12 (1985):458–461.

14. Escamillae RF et al. "Effects of Technique Variations on Knee Biomechanics during the Squat and Leg Press." *Med Sci Sports Exerc* 33 (2001):1552–1566.

15. American College of Sports Medicine. *Exercise Prescription & Testing,* 7th ed. (Baltimore, MD: Lippincott Williams & Wilkins, 2006).

16. Hicks JE, Joe GO, Gerber LH. "Rehabilitation of the Patient with Inflammatory Arthritis and Connective-Tissue Disease." In *Physical Medicine & Rehabilitation: Principles and Practice,* 4th ed. DeLisa, J ed. (Philadelphia, PA: Lippincott Williams & Wilkins, 2005), 781–785.

17. Machover S, Sapecky AJ. "Effect of Isometric Exercise on the Quadriceps Muscle in Patients with Rheumatoid Arthritis." *Arch Phys Med Rehabil* 47 (1966): 737–741.

18. "Rheumatoid Arthritis Center," www.mayoclinic.com (accessed Dec. 29, 2007).

11

EXERCISE AND OSTEOPOROSIS

Christopher Morin and Jennifer Morin

If you went into an exercise facility twenty years ago you would mostly find individuals looking to improve sports performance or their physical appearance. At the same time research emerged that received a tremendous amount of media attention, which altered fitness memberships from mostly young people to include middle aged and older individuals as well. Some of the exciting areas of research were in sacropeneia and osteoporosis prevention and treatment (see sacropeneia sidebar).

When it comes to osteoporosis weight bearing exercise, including resistance training, may increase and/or maintain bone mass while improving factors that may prevent fractures from falls, such as balance, muscle strength, and body weight. According to the American College of Sports Medicine (ACSM), exercise builds bone mass in children and adolescents, maintains or modestly builds bone in young adults, and assists in minimizing bone loss in older adults.[1] This means that while exercising may not build bone mass to a great degree in older people, there are still tremendous benefits—no matter what age they begin. Seniors should look to keeping the bone they have while the possibility of building bone is a bonus.

Keep in mind these two key points from the *Surgeon General's Report* (SGR) *on Bone Health and Osteoporosis:*

1. Weak bones should not just be excused as a natural part of aging.
2. People of all ages can improve their bone health.

WHAT IS OSTEOPOROSIS?

People need to be aware that osteoporosis is a bone disease. Being known as a disease and not a mere condition makes them stand up and notice. Known also as porous bone, it is characterized as low bone mass and structural deterioration of bone tissue. In other words the quantity and quality of bone is affected, which can make it fragile and more likely to break. Unfortunately

Sacropenia

The term "sacropenia" was first used over fifteen years ago in the landmark book *Biomarkers, the 10 Keys to Prolonging Vitality.*[16] Sacropenia refers to an overall weakening of the body caused by a gradual, decades-long change in body composition in favor of fat with loss of muscle mass. Dr. William Evans and Irwin Rosenberg who developed the term describe within *Biomarkers* two important studies done at their Tuft's University laboratories suggesting a decline in muscle strength and size is not an inevitable part of aging. Their colleague, Dr. Walter Frontera, found that older subjects, ages 60 to 72 years, were able to gain both strength and muscular size from weight training. Before this study other investigators did not push their subjects hard enough, usually having them train at 30 to 40 percent of 1 RM. Frontera's research group encouraged their subjects to train like younger people at 80 percent of 1 RM. After twelve consecutive weeks, three days a week, their efforts paid off with daily average increase in extensors and flexors strength of 3.3 and 6.5 percent and a 12 percent collective increase in muscle mass. The amount of muscle mass increase was what would be expected in younger people following the same regimen. A follow-up study by Dr. Maria Fiatrone at the same laboratory expanded on the past study by investigating the frail, institutionalized elderly, 87 to 96 years old. The findings were suggested to be even more startling, where subjects' muscle strength almost tripled and muscle size grew by 10 percent. The authors of *Biomarkers* and their Tuft's University colleagues were one of the first research groups to suggest that muscle mass and strength can be regained, no matter what your age and no matter what the state of your body musculature is before starting an exercise program. Therefore, strength training the elderly has become an essential part of their physical conditioning program and is regularly recommended by physicians and warranted by other health professionals.

the disease can act silently progressing painlessly until a bone fractures, which typically occurs in the hip, spine, and wrist, but other sites may be affected.

The most severe fracture is at the hip, which generally requires hospitalization and major surgery. It can impair a person's ability to walk unassisted and may cause prolonged or permanent disability or even death. Spinal or vertebral fractures also have serious consequences, including loss of height, severe back pain, and deformity. These fractures can occur with minimal trauma, in some cases there can be no trauma at all, where the act of standing up to walk can be the breaking point. In some cases where an individual falls and breaks a hip, the fall is not what breaks the hip it is the breaking of the hip that causes the fall.

Osteopenia is a term often heard these days in association with osteoporosis. It is not osteoporosis, but it's a precursor to it where bone density is below average (1.5 to 2.5 standard deviations below a young adult mean, while osteoporosis is 2.5 standard deviations below the mean). Osteopenia places one at a greater risk for osteoporosis and its related fractures. Having osteopenia does not mean you'll get osteoporosis, it puts you at higher risk. Luckily osteopenia and osteoporosis can be prevented, as well as diagnosed and treated.

WHO IS AFFECTED?

Osteoporosis affects all ethnic groups. The incidence is highest in Caucasion and Asian women, but occurs in other women and men too. Though some people think of osteoporosis as a disease of older individuals, in fact it can strike at any age. However, it's true that the risk increases with age. According to the SGR it is a major health threat in America impacting an estimated 44 million Americans, where 55 percent of the people over 50 years of age have it. In the United States, there are 10 million estimated to already have it with an additional 34 million at increased risk for osteoporosis due to low bone mass.[2]

Despite the television ads with the actress Sally Fields depicting osteoporosis as a disease affecting only women, both men and women can suffer from it. Although women are four times more likely than men to develop the disease, a statistic suggests that one out of every two women and one in four men over 50 will have a fracture from osteoporosis in their lifetime.

WHY ARE WOMEN MORE AFFECTED?

Although men can develop osteoporosis, 80 percent of those affected by osteoporosis are women. Women structurally have less bone tissue than men to start and lose bone faster due to the changes that happen with menopause. On average, men at the age of 50 start to experience a 0.4 percent per year loss of bone, while women dramatically start losing almost 1 percent at the age of 35. The loss of bone at this rate is typically not a problem for men until their eighties, but for women due to the increase rate of bone loss during menopause of up to 3 percent per year a 30 percent loss of bone mass by the age of 70 is not unusual.

HOW SERIOUS ARE OSTEOPOROTIC FRACTURES?

Osteoporosis is responsible for more than 1.5 million fractures annually, including 300,000 hip fractures, approximately 700,000 vertebral fractures, 250,000 wrist fractures, and more than 300,000 fractures at other sites. An average of 24 percent of hip fracture patients aged 50 and over die in the year following their fracture. At six months after a hip fracture, only 15 percent of hip fracture patients can walk across a room unaided. Many who have suffered a hip fracture feel isolated, depressed, or afraid to leave home because they fear falling, which can lead to further disability. The rate of hip fractures is two to three times higher in women than men. The one year mortality following a hip fracture is nearly twice as high for men as for women. Unfortunately in case of a hip fractures women are at a fourfold greater risk of a second one.

Based on data the estimated expense for osteoporosis and related fractures ranges from $14 to $18 billion each year. The SGR suggest that the cost of a hip fracture for one individual can be more than $81,000 during his or her lifetime. Considering all of these statistics osteoporosis is a serious health problem.

WHAT ARE THE RISK FACTORS FOR OSTEOPOROSIS?

The loss of bone mass has been linked with physical inactivity, hormonal, nutritional, mechanical, and genetic factors. As with many of the diseases discussed within this text, osteoporosis can be debilitating affecting one's quality of life and ability to remain independent. Osteoporosis has many risk factors associated to its development—some are modifiable through lifestyle changes while others are not. An interesting point is that many with the osteoporosis have several risk factors, but others may have none. Another key point is that certain groups and people are more likely to develop osteoporosis than others are. You should determine what risk factors you have for both heart disease and osteoporosis; finding out your status is a must thing to do.

Osteoporosis Risk Factors

Non-modifiable

Advanced age
Family history of osteoporosis
A past fracture after age 50
Ethnicity (Caucasian and Asian women are at highest risk)

Potentially Modifiable

Being small and thin
Low bone mass (osteopenia)
Abnormal absence of menstrual periods (amenorrhea)
Anorexia nervosa
Estrogen deficiency as a result of menopause
Low testosterone level in men
Inactive lifestyle
Calcium deficiency
Vitamin D deficiency
Medications (corticosteroids, chemotherapy, anticonvulsants)
Smoking
Excessive use of alcohol

What Happens to Bone as We Age?

Bones are truly an amazing structure where some can withstand several times a person's body weight, but they are not indestructible. To understand osteoporosis we should look at what happens with a bone as we age. Bone is living tissue. It is made up of proteins that make up a lattice and calcium salt that adds strength and hardness to the protein framework. These compounds give the bone flexibility and strength.

As with other body tissues old parts are removed and new parts are formed—this is known as *resorption* and *formation*. During one's early years, new bone formation is faster than resorption resulting in bones becoming larger and denser. This occurs until approximately age 30; thereafter resorption slowly begins to be greater than bone formation. Some suggest that by the age 20 the average woman has acquired 98 percent of her skeletal mass.

Studies suggest that greater than 75 percent of U.S. adults don't consume the recommended amount of calcium, where 25 percent of women get less than a third of the recommended amount.[3] This results in the body drawing calcium from the body through its reserve found in bone. If this continues osteopenia develops, and if prolonged osteoporosis, especially if optimal peak bone mass is not reached during younger bone-building years. Bone loss is especially found in women going through the first few years of menopause. The increased rate of bone loss during menopause is linked to a decrease in estrogen production. The protection provided by estrogen is not clear, but some individuals use estrogen replacement to combat osteoporosis. This therapy is considered dramatic due its association with cancer of the uterus and breast.

Therefore, building strong bones during childhood and adolescence is suggested to be the best defense against developing osteoporosis later in life. Children and teens should get at least one hour of physical activity every day. Recommended activities are somewhat high impact and weight bearing such as jumping rope, running, and playing sports.

What Are the Symptoms of Osteoporosis?

Osteoporosis is often called a "silent disease" due to no apparent symptoms or signs for bone loss. Often the first clue that one has this condition is a bone fracture. However, there may be other clues such as loss of height, back pain, and kyphosis (stooped posture), which can occur from collapsed vertebrae.

Loss of strength impacts quality of life and has been suggested to be a possible marker for osteoporosis.[3,4] Research has shown that postmenopausal women without osteoporosis were up to 20 percent stronger dynamically than their osteoporotic counterparts. Some have suggested the use of dynamic strength tests as screening tool for osteoporosis. A study by Sinaki et al. described a negative association between back extensor strength and both kyphosis and number of vertebral fractures—the authors noted that increasing back strength may prove to be an effective therapeutic intervention for the osteoporotic spine.[5]

Doctors usually look for osteoporosis using a bone mineral density (BMD) test, which can measure bone density in various sites of the body. The most widely recognized bone mineral density test is called a dual-energy x-ray absorptiometry or DXA test. This test is safe, painless, and doesn't take much time (ten minutes or less). It can detect osteoporosis before a fracture occurs and possibly predict fractures in the future. Testing on a regular basis is done to determine rate of bone loss and to see if treatments are effective. Luckily, the combination of treatment and testing has been found to be associated with a decrease in hip fracture occurrence. According to the SGR, all women over 65 and anyone who has a bone fracture after age 50 should get a bone density test. Others with significant risk factors should also get a bone density test as well.

TREATMENT OF OSTEOPOROSIS

There are two types of interventions used to reduce the risk of osteoportic fracture, nonpharmacologic and pharmacological. Nonpharmacologic interventions include calcium and vitamin D supplementation, fall prevention education, weight-bearing exercise, balance training, and muscle building. Pharmacological options are the bisphosphonates, estrogen therapy, raloxifene, and the anabolic agent teriparatide. According to Levine regardless of what treatment regimen is selected, health care providers need to emphasize the importance of compliance and adherence to improve persistence with therapy, and subsequent fracture reduction efficacy.[6]

Considering that this is an exercise text, a discussion of calcium and vitamin D supplementation, fall prevention education, and pharmacological agents is beyond its scope. It must be stressed that the recommendations made for osteoporosis prevention are different for its treatment, therefore if you have osteoporosis already, talk to your doctor about what you should be doing to treat this condition.

EXERCISE AND PREVENTION OF OSTEOPOROSIS

Active people of all ages have greater bone mass compared to their inactive peers. This disparity continues as one ages into one's seventies and eighties. Therefore it is wise to be active throughout life. Exercises that are weight bearing seem to be the best at maintaining bone, where stress is placed along the long axis of the bone. How you exercise can influence where bone density is the strongest. For example, walking briskly may build bone in the hips and thighs but it does not build bone in the wrist. This is clearly seen in studies of athletes such as tennis and baseball players, who have increased bone mass in their dominant arms compared to their nondominant arms.

The amount of exercise needed for bone development seems to be related to the magnitude of force and the frequency of application as well as the aforementioned point of application. Past prevailing theory suggests that bone formation is caused by mechanical stress being converted to an electric signal that stimulates bone-building cells (osteoblasts). The mechanical stress has to be of a sufficient magnitude. The term minimal essential strain has been used to depict the threshold needed, in other words sufficient magnitude, for new bone formation. The magnitude of force needed to build new bone is above normal daily activities and is relative to each individual. For someone who is young, the minimal essential strain could be running, while for someone older or sedentary, brisk walking could surpass the threshold. Thus, it's a relative threshold—what works for one person may not for another. The question also arises of what is more important—load (resistance training) or frequency, repetition of movement (walking, jogging).[7] An analysis by Block et al. of active men compared to sedentary controls found men who lifted weights had the highest bone density values among active men.[8]

Research has shown that increases in the size and strength of muscle is correlated with an increase in bone mass, and vice versa, where a decrease in the size and strength of muscle is correlated with a decrease in bone mass. Loss of bone from young adulthood to the age of 80 is comparable to the strength loss of 35 to 40 percent during the same period. Therefore, a discussion on how to build muscle *and* strength is paramount. Simple bone building marker outside of a sophisticated test is increase in muscle size and strength. Fitness professionals use simple circumference measures and strength tests as a guide.

People who train regularly understand that building muscle takes weeks of training, unfortunately ceasing conditioning just for a couple of weeks will cause dramatic muscular changes. Therefore it's not worth taking off a substantial amount of time from training. The same is true for bone. Bone formation takes a much longer time than bone resorption. This is seen clearly from bed rest studies where bone loss occurs rapidly from only a few weeks of bed rest and from the observations of astronauts who have actually broken bones trying to walk after long space missions. From these studies muscular contractions seem to be less important than weight bearing. One study found that just three hours a day of nonactive standing preserved spine bone mass. Therefore the National Strength and Conditioning Association (NSCA) recommends loading the spine through a weight-bearing force when trying to build bone.[9] Other authorities agree that weight-bearing activities that place additional stress to the stress of one's body weight seem to be the most effective.

The guideline from the NSCA as well as other authorities is to build up bone mass to peak levels as a child and early adult through high-loading weight-bearing exercises and sports, such as gymnastics, volleyball, and basketball. These activities have been shown to increase bone density at what is termed clinically relevant sites like the hip and spine compared to lower intensity activities. Similar type activities like running, squash, tennis, and some types of aerobic class seem to fall within this category.

The exercise recommendation within this section applies to healthy, asymptomatic individuals free of disease. As discussed throughout this text aerobic

What Is the Difference between Exercise and Physical Activity?

Before we move on I need to address the difference between the terms exercise and physical activity. They are sometimes used interchangeably, but as worded in research studies they are quite different. Physical activity encompasses all human movement, most notably activities of daily living, while exercise is considered planned physical activity with the goal of increasing fitness. Planned exercise, or sometimes termed formal exercise, is rhythmic and continuous movement. A majority of people are recommended to do it at a moderate intensity most days a week for twenty to thirty minutes, like walking at a brisk pace. Physical activity in addition to formal exercise is also recommended, such as those extra caloric-burning movements of say climbing flights of stairs instead of an elevator or parking a greater distance from an entrance or raking leaves. Increases in physical activity and formal exercise can improve health and fitness, but formal exercise is superior in developing physical capacity. Both formal exercise and increasing daily physical activity should be part of an osteoporosis prevention program. Due to the difficulty of regulating activities of daily living, increasing physical activity as a treatment for osteoporosis should be scrutinized as well secondary to formal exercise in the treatment of osteoporosis.

exercise is extremely important for health and well-being. To improve aerobic capacity a certain threshold should be met. Typically individuals use heart rate to determine that level, where the heart rate reserve (HRR) equation is used (see HRR equation in Chapter 9). When it comes to prevention of osteoporosis through aerobic exercise follow ACSM guidelines for healthy people of three to five days per week, at 50 to 85 percent HRR, for twenty to thirty minutes. Aerobic exercises have limits in their ability to increase bone mass due to one's aerobic ability and body weight. The NSCA suggests interval training or to wear a weight vest or using hand weights as a way to further increase bone mass through aerobic activities.

The NSCA and ACSM recommend resistance training for building bone and for the prevention and treatment of osteoporosis. The NSCA suggests that studies of resistance training on bone formation have been variable; some have showed significant results while others have not. It seems that the studies that showed no increases have not been intense enough or offered exercises that were specific for bone building. The choice of exercises suggested by the NSCA should involve motions that use multiple muscle groups that direct forces through the spine and hips. Termed structural exercises, they include squats, lunge, push presses, cleans, deadlifts for the lower body and bench presses and shoulder presses for the upper body. Other exercises that fit this criteria are the leg press machine, plate loaded hack and leg press, stability ball squats with weight or one leg at a time, and squats and lunges using a functional trainer. Use of muscle isolation exercises, like weight training machines (Nautilus, Cybex, etc.), has possibly less of a bone-building effect and therefore should be limited or used in association with other structural, weight-bearing exercises. For example, instead of using a leg extension machine alone, use structural exercises like the squat instead of or in addition to this machine.

As with resistance training to build stronger and bigger muscles, progressively increase loads to increase bone as, similar to muscle, bone gets accustomed to the same loads. When conditioning stays the same, which is referred to as *maintenance*, equilibrium is reached and bone and muscle mass will stay the same until the training becomes progressive. It's important to avoid injury and to not take on too much of a load when participating in strength training. Allow enough time for recovery between exercise sessions for bone and muscle remodeling. This will help avoid overuse injuries like stress fractures and tendonitis—at least forty-eight hours is typically recommended between resistance training sessions. The NSCA also recommends changing the distribution of forces by using a variety of resistance exercises in order to present unique stimuli to the bone and to avoid overuse injury.

In summary, the NSCA suggests several training keys for bone building; specificity of loading, progressive overload, exercise variation, and weight bearing. The number of sets per exercise suggested by the NSCA is three to six at no more than ten repetitions, where each set ends with momentary muscular fatigue. As mentioned, structural exercises should be the cornerstone of the program.

I like to point out an important resistance training statement by the ACSM. As with aerobic training, resistance training must have an overload for adaptation to occur. The overload must surpass a minimal threshold for strength development. High intensity training at or near maximal effort is the greatest stimuli. The ACSM notes that development is not just about the *amount of weight* it is also concerned with the *quality of motion*. Changing one of the following variables can increase intensity:

- Increasing weight or resistance
- Increasing the number of repetitions
- Reducing speed of movement (reducing momentum)
- Avoiding locking out at the top of motions, like presses, keeps tension on the muscle

Ironically, some studies show that lower repetitions seem to better increase bone density in older populations. Bone density seems to increase more with lower reps (seven to ten) versus higher (fourteen to eighteen). Those at risk for osteoporosis or who have osteopenia are advised by the ACSM to train at lower reps with high intensity. It's also important to have a variety of exercises that impose stress from different angles.

It is very important to begin or advance an exercise program with the help of professionals in order to avoid injury and prevent other health problems. Qualified supervision should be used in instructing correct technique and before increasing loads and employing structural exercises. Isolation exercises, like the weight training machines, are a great place to start introducing people to resistance training. This introduction, which may last several weeks, will build a solid foundation before moving to more challenging structural exercises. It must be stressed that when training with structural exercises correct execution is mandatory before increasing loads.

EXERCISE AND TREATMENT OF OSTEOPOROSIS

If you have osteopenia or osteoporosis talk to your doctor about an appropriate exercise program. Often testing should be done before starting an exercise program in many cases. In some situations older individuals should have a graded exercise test before starting a vigorous exercise program. In those with osteoporosis a physician approval is recommended before graded exercise testing to determine the risk to benefit ratio. When testing is recommended an upright posture should be maintained at all times, where the avoidance of spinal flexion is important to avoid stressing vulnerable vertebrae. The use of a cycle ergometer is preferred testing device over a treadmill. The technician should be aware that osteoportic pain may terminate the test before reaching testing thresholds. Severe kyphosis (stooped posture), due to multiple vertebrae fractures, may compromise ventilatory capacity and shift forward an individual's center of gravity. Treadmill testing is not preferred but if used safety must be stressed at all times. Additional tests recommended by the ACSM include balance, muscular strength, and gait biomechanics.

Many of the concepts discussed for the prevention of osteoporosis apply to the treatment of osteoporosis, but certain safety considerations must be taken. After testing is completed some of the same recommendations for testing should be employed while exercising, such as an upright posture should be maintained at all times and the avoidance of spinal flexion and osteoportic pain. For those who are not severely limited by pain the following exercise recommendations generally apply. Remember for those who are severely limited by pain consult a physician before exercise participation.

The ACSM recommends osteoportic individuals to perform cardiovascular exercise (aquatic, walking, cycling) at 40 to 70 percent of HRR. Although aquatic exercise is not highly recommended in the prevention of osteoporosis, it is for the treatment of osteoporosis for it is typically safe and well tolerated, especially in individuals who can not tolerate weight bearing due to arthritic or osteoportic pain. Aquatic exercises, like swimming, do not build bone density to the same degree as weight bearing activities like walking or running, but may contribute to building bone due to the high intensity muscular activity that they require. Weight bearing aerobic exercise, like vigorous walking, is recommended for those who don't have pain. Aerobic exercise should be performed four or more days per week for twenty or more minutes. It's fine to limit this to up to forty-five minutes in order to avoid injury, while splitting sessions into five- or ten-minute bouts in order to build up to twenty or more minutes is generally acceptable. Using hand weights and wearing a weighted vest as suggested in the prevention section is not recommended in the treatment of osteoporosis.

Balance and functional exercises are highly recommended, especially considering vertebrae fractures may shift an individual's center of gravity forward. Simple standing on one leg without support is a great place to begin balance training, thereafter when this is mastered one can move on to using a balance device. Always have a support available when beginning balance training. Functional exercise are simple motions that duplicate activities of daily living like getting up from a floor, or out of a chair, or climbing a fight of stairs, or reaching overhead into a cabinet (see chapter 6).

As with the prevention of osteoporosis, resistance training can be used in osteoporosis treatment. The ACSM recommends resistance exercises (free weights, weight machines, calisthenics, and elastic bands) that direct forces over the long axis of the bone. Typically training should be two days per week where each exercise is performed for eight to ten repetitions at submaximal intensities for one or two sets. Again, all exercises should be performed without spinal flexion with an upright posture. Some of the structural exercises as suggested in the prevention section can be modified or used in the treatment of osteoporosis, but only cautiously and with qualified supervision (such as squats with dumbbells and the seated leg press machine); the previously mentioned weight training machines is a great place to start introducing osteporotic individuals to resistance training. As always, avoid an exercise if there is pain.

Sports that employ explosive movements and high impact loading, like running and jumping, should not be performed (examples are tennis, basketball, volleyball). Other sports like golf and daily physical activities that require excessive bending at the waist or twisting should be avoided due to high spinal compressive forces and the increased vulnerability to fracture. Unfortunately just sitting and bending may cause a fracture in those suffering from osteoporosis.

BACK CARE AND OSTEOPOROSIS

Considering the importance of proper posture and exercise body positions on spinal care for those with and without osteoporosis further elaboration is warranted. Stuart McGill, a renowned authority on low back health, suggests fully flexing the spine repeatedly or being in a fully flexed position for a prolonged period of time may cause disc herniation.[10] He goes further to suggest that disc herniation is almost impossible with out full spinal flexion. He suggests that some low back machines, which isolate lumbar motion by extension against a resistance pad from full flexion to neutral, might promote disc herniation. Care must be taken if using this type of machine, where range of motion should be limited, the spine should never be flexed, and back extension must be kept at all times. Other exercises that might be harmful are full sit-ups, spinal flexion stretches, and exercises where the lumbar spine may become fully flexed. Considering spinal flexion may occur to a degree during most exercises, care must be taken when performing any exercise. Furthermore, lumbar posture should be kept in a neutral position while performing exercises and activities of daily living. Avoid twisting against resistance as well.

Flexibility training is often recommended as part of a fitness regimen. The ACSM recommends that it should be part of a program for people with osteoporosis. McGill suggests that spine flexibility should not be emphasized with low back disorders until the spine has stabilized and has undergone strength and endurance training and in some cases the patient may never reach this stage. McGill also notes that there is little data to support that a major emphasis on flexibility will improve back health and lessen the risk of injury. People with osteoporosis should avoid stretches that flex the spine, while other stretches that do not are acceptable.

Simple home-based, low-intensity, floor exercises can be effective treatment for those with osteoporosis. In a study by Hongo et al. osteoprotic subjects were instructed to lift their upper trunk from a prone position and maintain the neutral position over several repetitions, after several weeks of training there was an improvement in quality of life and back extensor strength.[11] Other simple exercises that one can usually do quite safely include supine bridges, side-bridges on knees, and planks on knees (each position is held for five seconds and repeated for ten repetitions for one to two sets). Another home-based trunk strengthening program by Chien et al. showed improved trunk mobility and strength and enhanced quality of life in osteoporotic and osteopenic postmenopausal women without vertebral fracture.[12] As mentioned, thoracic kyphosis (stooped posture) has been suggested as a marker for osteoporosis, while in the past it was thought as a natural, nonreversible process of aging. A study by Itoi and Sinaki suggests that increasing the back extensor strength in healthy estrogen-deficient women helps decrease thoracic kyphosis.[13] In treating kyphosis the row motion with bands and free weights seem very beneficial.

Mostly everyone can benefit from simple home-based spinal exercises to avoid injury, disease, and to improve functional ability.

In conclusion, something needs to be done about osteoporosis. The SGR suggests that if immediate action is not taken, half of all Americans over 50 will have weak bones from osteoporosis and low bone mass by 2020. This could cause the number of hip fractures in the United States to double or even triple by 2040.

Americans need to become physically active every day. As of now more than half of all Americans do not get enough physical activity to build bones. Regular exercise is vital for health and well-being, especially as we age. In older individuals, a setback in their physical activity due to lack of motivation, injury, or fracture can lead to disuse, which leads to less function and further debilitation.

If you are overwhelmed by all the recommendations just try walking for ten to thirty minutes; brisk walking most days of the weeks is a great exercise and has far-reaching health benefits. This exercise will not only help to keep your bones healthy, it will improve your health overall. Even joint health can be improved as joints need to be moved on a regular basis so that cartilage, meniscus, and other structures can be nourished, which wards off arthritis and other disorders of the joint.

Individuals concerned about osteoporosis also need to focus on proper nutrition and safety, especially in trying to prevent fracture producing falls. One study by Swanenburg et al. found an 89 percent reduction in falls reported in the experimental group receiving multiple interventions.[14] If you are at risk or have osteoporosis, consult with your physician about the types of interventions such as dietary strategies, exercises, and medications that have been shown to slow or stop bone loss. There are many safety steps that you can take in your house or outside to prevent a fall as well.

Muscle and bone adapt to the stresses presented to them; simply put, they get stronger when stressed and weaker when not. Remember the old maxim, "If you don't use it you will lose it." Alarming research data from the Framingham Disability found that a significant amount of women over 55 were unable to lift just 10 pounds, which must limit one's ability to perform daily tasks.[15] Exercise with the goal of increasing function and independence look at an improvement in tone and shape as a bonus.

REFERENCES

1. *ACSM's Guidelines for Exercise Testing and Prescription,* 7th ed. (2006). Baltimore, MD: Lippincott, Williams, & Wilkins.

2. U.S. Department of Health and Human Services. *Bone Health and Osteoporosis: A Report of the Surgeon General.* Washington, DC: U.S. Department of Health and Human Services, Office of the Surgeon General, 2004.

3. McArdle WD, Katch FI, Katch VL. *Exercise Physiology: Energy, Nutrition, and Human Performance.* 3rd ed. Malvern, PA: Lea & Febiger, 1991.

4. Miyakoshi N, Hongo M, Maekawa S, Ishikawa Y, Shimada Y, Itoi E. Back extensor strength and lumbar spinal mobility are predictors of quality of life in patients with postmenopausal osteoporosis. *Osteoporos Int* 18 (2007):1397–1403.

5. Sinaki M, Wollan PC, Scott RW, Gelczer RK. Can strong back extensors prevent vertebral fractures in women with osteoporosis? *Mayo Clin Proc* 71 (1996):951–956.

6. Levine JP. Pharmacologic and nonpharmacologic management of osteoporosis. *Clin Cornerstone* 8 (2006):40–53.

7. Snow-Harter C, Marcus R. *Exercise, Bone Mineral Density, and Osteoporosis. Exercise and Sports Sciences Reviews.* Volume 19. ACSM. Philadelphia, PA: Williams & Wilkins, 1991.

8. Block JE, Genant HK, Black D. Greater vertebral bone density in exercising young men. *West J Med* 145 (1986):39–42.

9. Baechle, E (ed). *Essential of Strength and Conditioning.* 2nd ed. National Strength and Conditioning Association. Champaign, IL: Human Kinetics, 2000.

10. McGill S. *Low Back Disorders: Evidence Based Prevention and Rehabilitation.* Champaign, IL: Human Kinetics, 2002.

11. Hongo M, Itoi E, Sinaki M, et al. Effect of low-intensity back exercise on quality of life and back extensor strength in patients with osteoporosis: a randomized controlled trial. *Osteoporos Int* 18 (2007):1389–1395.

12. Chien MY, Yang RS, Tsauo JY. Home-based trunk-strengthening exercise for osteoporotic and osteopenic postmenopausal women without fracture—a pilot study. *Clin Rehabil* 19 (2005):579.

13. Itoi E, Sinaki M. Effect of back-strengthening exercise on posture in healthy women 49 to 65 years of age. *Mayo Clin Proc* 69 (1994):1054–1059.

14. Swanenburg J, de Bruin ED, Stauffacher M, Mulder T, Uebelhart D. Effects of exercise and nutrition on postural balance and risk of falling in elderly people with decreased bone mineral density: Randomized controlled trial pilot study. *Clin Rehabil.* 21 (2007):523–534.

15. Jette A, Branch L. The Framingham Disability Study II: Physical disability among the aging. *Am J Public Health* 71 (1981):1211–1216.

16. Evans W, Rosenberg I. *Biomarkers; the 10 Keys to Prolonging Vitality.* New York: Fireside, Simon and Schuster, 1992.

12

EXERCISE AND FIBROMYALGIA

Kim Dupree Jones, Janice H. Hoffman, and Diane G. Adams

Exercise is a vital component of a comprehensive treatment plan for people with fibromyalgia (FM).[1] FM is a multisymptomatic disorder defined by a history of widespread pain and specified tender points.[2] However, most people with FM are multisymptomatic with stiffness, fatigue, disrupted sleep, back pain, cognitive dysfunction and overexertion-induced symptom flares.[3] FM, like many chronic illnesses, may be associated with a genetic predisposition. This genetic predisposition may be triggered by environment insults such as head and neck trauma from a motor vehicle accident, prolonged viral illness, a persistent regional pain, or unremitting stress. FM affects 7 percent of the adult female population and costs an estimated \$20 billion annually.[3-5]

It is imperative to provide evidence-based exercise advice to maximize treatment effectiveness. The purpose of this chapter is to review FM clinical trials on exercise, provide a rational approach for gentle, progressive exercise, and explain how to minimize the kinds of physical activities that often result in a symptom flare.

THE RESEARCH

History of Exercise Studies and FM

At one time, bed rest was the most common prescription for any person experiencing pain, whether the pain was acute or chronic. However, the role of bed rest versus exercise in chronic pain conditions is more complex. Too much exercise can result in a symptom flare, while too little over time can cause deconditioning and a cycle of increased disability.

The first consideration of exercise as potentially therapeutic occurred in a landmark 1975 sleep trial. To investigate the relationship between sleep and pain, Moldofsky and colleagues repeatedly startled sleeping college students awake shortly after they entered a deep sleep cycle. This manipulation resulted in muscle pain in the majority of subjects, while surprisingly sparing the few students who were elite runners.[6,7] This forwarded the notion that sleep is essential to well-being, and further, that physical exercise might play a role in helping to mitigate pain.

In 1988, McCain and colleagues were the first to conduct a randomized controlled trial of exercise in FM.[8] Two subject groups exercised, the first group performing aerobic endurance training on a stationary bike, while the control group performed simple flexibility training. Although the aerobic endurance group experienced hip/buttock pain, their program prompted enhanced physical conditioning.

McCain's study demonstrated that aerobic activity could benefit those with FM by avoiding deconditioning, even if the exercise did not significantly improve sleep or pain. His data provided an important paradigm shift: People with FM can maintain fitness and function through exercise. Instead of extended rest, clinicians could confidently prescribe a program that included exercise as part of the total treatment plan.

Over the next two decades, forty-six FM exercise interventions with a total enrollment of 3,035 FM subjects took place. The goal was to determine the optimal frequency, intensity, length, and type of exercise for symptomatic relief and fitness improvements in FM. Results from these studies indicate that many types of exercise are beneficial: Land-based and pool-based cardio training, strength training, flexibility training, T'ai Chi, and QiGong. Gentle exercise combined with balneotherapy (mineral baths) and thalassotherapy (use of sea-based spa treatments) proved beneficial for symptom relief as well.[9]

It became clear through these studies that the key difference between success and failure in an FM exercise prescription was the intensity and frequency of exercise. Unfortunately, those trials consistent with guidelines recommended by the U.S. Surgeon General for healthy individuals often resulted in a worsening of FM symptoms, which in turn led to high study attrition rates. However, research trials that offered lower heart rate intensities, less impact activities (e.g., walking instead of running or jumping) were tolerated and almost universally improved functional fitness, defined as exercise that prepares the body to perform daily activities, such as bending down, lifting objects, or climbing stairs, without injury or discomfort.

Overall, well-informed FM exercise interventions do appear to be effective at reducing fatigue, disrupted sleep, and easing tight muscles, although there are mixed results related to pain improvement. A gap remains in the literature regarding symptom and fitness improvement in studies involving combination drug and exercise trials, despite how common this protocol is in clinical practice. Some FM researchers promote the idea that adequate symptom management increases the likelihood of exercise success.[10,11]

Risk versus Benefit of Exercise in FM

When someone with FM has becomes deconditioned, it might appear to him or her that even the simplest of movements can cause an increase in pain. Adding exercise as a treatment therapy would naturally seem counterproductive.

Fear of a symptom flare is quite rational when prior exercise sessions have brought on DOMS (Delayed Onset Muscle Soreness).

DOMS is pain or discomfort that peaks twenty-four to seventy-two hours after exercising and generally subsides within two to three days. Once thought to be brought on by lactic acid buildup, a more comprehensive theory is that it is caused by tiny tears in the muscle fibers caused by repetitive eccentric contractions or unaccustomed activity or training levels. DOMS can occur in anyone when muscles are overtaxed.

However, in FM the muscle microtrauma of DOMS does not repair quickly and symptoms may be more severe and may continue beyond the typical two- to three-day range. This lack of normal repair in FM is likely due to a lack of quality sleep common in FM, and/or low levels of a growth hormone called IGF-1.[12]

In summary, the most natural response to movement-caused pain is exercise avoidance. It is crucial those with FM be informed that exercise, when performed with FM-specific modifications, will not automatically increase pain or fatigue levels. Further, they need to know they can exercise all muscles, even those that hurt. These patients can be reassured that no permanent muscle or joint damage occurs during appropriate exercise.

In fact, just the opposite is true: The body requires movement to stay supple and maintain the strength needed for activities of daily living. Conditioned muscles in proper alignment are pliable, which gives the body fluid mobility and lessens "fatigue posture" pain. When muscles are not used, they become tight; and inflexible, stiff muscle fibers pull on ligaments and tendons, which are rich with pain-sensing nerve fibers.[13] So in fact, exercise is essential for avoiding a cycle leading to increased disability, as shown in Figure 12.1.

Now that researchers agree exercising improves physical function, quality of sleep, and fatigue in the majority of FM subjects, the question becomes "how does someone with FM optimally begin an exercise program?"

THE EXERCISE PRESCRIPTION—AN OVERVIEW

Those who have been sedentary for more than three months should never jump into a vigorous daily regime right away. Exercise can help control pain in the long term, but if a fibromyalgia symptom flare is present, it is best to wait and begin exercise after the pain subsides. Once symptoms of a flare are in remission, a gradual progression into gentle exercise can begin.[14]

Persons with FM who maintained a very active lifestyle before their condition took hold may want to "make up for lost time" when pain symptoms are improved. They can easily overwork, causing the cycle of pain, recovery, overexertion, and pain shown in Figure 12.1. This defeats the overall goal of decreasing pain levels in the long term. Initially, the beginning exerciser with FM should walk away from each session feeling they could have done more instead of feeling they went to their limit. This is because the ultimate goal is not

Figure 12.1
Negative Physical Exertion Cycle in Fibromyalgia

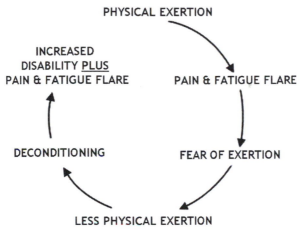

Source: © JH Hoffman and KD Jones 2007. Courtesy of Kim Jones.

elite athletic fitness, but rather the creation of a stronger body, capable of moving through the activities of daily living without undue stress or increased pain levels.

There are five main progression steps for FM. They include:

1. Corrected breathing technique
2. Restored postural alignment
3. Flexibility training
4. Strength training
5. Aerobic endurance training

No matter the current level of activity, progressing step-by-step through this order of body reconditioning will, over the long term, decrease pain and fatigue while increasing energy and quality of life.

Relearning proper breathing is the first step. Chronic pain can cause breath holding and reduced chest expansion. Removing obstructed breathing patterns is an essential start toward activities that will require increased oxygen. We will cover how to correct breathing patterns in the next section.

Good postural alignment is also crucial. With fibromyalgia, there are often taut bands of muscle around tender points. Muscles that remain short and tight hold the body in "pain postures" that need to be corrected before adding movement. This will give the body a solid foundation for the exercises to come. A description for finding good alignment follows below. Additionally, an excellent DVD showing neutral alignment positioning is available at www.myalgia.com.

Flexibility and strength training will get the body fit and able to function properly. This type of exercise goes hand in hand toward increasing a sense of well-being.

Regarding popular Pilates and yoga fitness class formats, the authors urge caution for those with FM. When postures or poses are held longer than ten seconds at a time, a deconditioned FM participant's muscles can quickly be overworked. Nonetheless, the back pain that is present in 100 percent of FM patients is minimized with core strengthening. The deep breathing and body awareness in many styles of yoga are also beneficial for FM. One-to-one instruction with an informed instructor would make the difference in this instance. The next section covers both flexibility and strength exercise routines. The combination of flexibility and strength, particularly in the hips, knees, and ankles may reduce falls and balance perturbations in people with FM.[15,16]

Key exercise recommendations for people with FM (versus traditional flexibility and strength training) include:

Never holding a stretch or strength pose over ten seconds

Minimizing eccentric strength movements (where the muscle lengthens against resistance)

Eliminating overhead movements and movements that keep the limbs away from the midline for extended periods

Avoiding repetitive motion by alternating limbs, changing the movement pattern frequently, and building in rest periods

A much more gradual timeline for training program level progressions

Aerobic endurance training includes walking, swimming, water aerobics, and low-intensity/low-impact aerobic dance. One critical goal of aerobic exercise is to build a strong heart. With a stronger heart, the body begins to pump blood more efficiently into the muscles, which will add capillaries that help the muscles manage longer workloads. The net result is endurance, that is, a body that can move for longer periods without fatigue.

Pacing is another consideration for those with FM.[17,18] Endurance needs to build very gradually. At first, it is reasonable to take time between aerobic activities by exercising in three five-minute bouts spread throughout the day. The long-term goal will be one twenty + minute period of aerobic endurance exercise three to four times per week.

For those with FM, endurance workouts that last longer than thirty minutes are generally not necessary and may increase the potential for delayed onset muscle soreness.[19,20] Additionally, taking a day off between endurance workouts gives FM muscles adequate time to repair.

Fibromyalgia Exercise Prescription I

The goal for a beginning exerciser with FM is to improve mobility without causing an increase in pain beyond the typical soreness felt when unused muscles begin working again.

For anyone who has been inactive, beginning to exercise again after more than three months of inactivity can be a teeth-gritting experience. For those with chronic pain and a proven potential for exercise-induced pain, the best starting point will be eliminating breathing disorders and gently realigning the body back to good posture, via flexibility adjustments dedicated to improving healthy body alignment.

Progression Step 1—Corrected Breathing Technique

Breath delivers oxygen to the body, which is a key component in aerobic metabolism. The heart then pumps oxygenated blood to skeletal muscles to aid in energy production. The diaphragm is the main "breathing" muscle. At each breath in, the diaphragm floats downward to allow the lungs to expand. On exhalation, the diaphragm rises, forcing air out of the lungs. The abdominal muscles are prepared to assist as well by moving inward as we exhale.

Chronic "pain postures" typically include high shoulders and a concave chest. Tight shoulder and chest musculature can produce the following restricted breathing patterns[21]:

Reverse breathing—where the abdomen moves out on exhalation and in on inhalation. This is the reverse of correct functional breathing.

Chest breathing—where the abdomen does no work and the diaphragm muscle does not fully rise or descend.

Collapsed breathing—where breathing is restricted to the upper chest. The lower lung area does not move during inhalation and the diaphragm muscle does not rise. A stomach bulge often occurs with this breathing pattern, along with a forward hunch to the shoulders.

Frozen breathing—is very shallow breathing, with no noticeable movement in the ribcage, abdomen, or back.

The solution to disordered breathing involves releasing muscular tension enough so that the abdomen will expand on inhalation and release toward the spine on exhalation.

The F.I.T. Prescription

Frequency: Practice this breathwork for at least four sessions per day until it becomes automatic

Intensity: None—the goal is to relax the body so this pattern becomes normal

Time: Approximately two to five minutes per session

Progression Step 2—Restored Postural Alignment

As mentioned above, chronic "pain postures" often include high shoulders, a head forward position, and a concave chest. They also include shortened, tight hip and thigh muscles, likely caused by prolonged sitting.

Good alignment includes the following:

The body's weight is supported at the center point of the feet
The legs at the knees are straight but not locked
The tailbone points down, but a natural curve remains in the low back
The ribcage floats over the pelvis with enough space for good breathing
The shoulders are back and down, away from the ears
The head sits tall on the neck with ears directly over shoulders

The F.I.T. Prescription

Frequency: Practice this postural alignment work at least two times per day until
    it feels natural
Intensity: Minimal—however, plan to continue holding the body in this optimal
    posture while moving through the day's tasks
Time: Approximately five to eight minutes

Progression Step 3—Flexibility Training

A flexibility training program focuses on lengthening short muscles. Our modern lifestyle has provided soft sofas and chairs and the ability to perform many more tasks while seated; this is true for the general population, not just those with FM. Consequently, the following muscles that typically need to be stretched tend to be tight from inactivity or from sitting for long periods:

Tight neck and upper back (the splenius, mastoids, and trapezius)
Tight front of shoulders (the anterior deltoids)
Tight chest (the pectorals)
Tight hips and backside (the IT band and piriformis)
Tight front of thighs (the iliopsoas and quadriceps)
Tight back of thighs (the hamstrings)
Tight calves (the gastrocnemius and soleus)
Tight insteps (the plantar fascia)

The F.I.T. Prescription

Frequency: For physical fitness and function, train for flexibility once daily. For
    reduction of pain and stiffness, a physical or occupational therapist may rec-
    ommend more frequent, shorter, less intense stretching of specified muscle
    groups based on symptom patterns and postures.
Intensity: Never bounce or overstretch. Move to the point of gentle resistance
    and hold.
Time: Hold each flexibility pose no longer than ten seconds. This daily training
    will take approximately fifteen to twenty minutes.

Progression Step 4—Strength Training

With the better postural support gained by the above flexibility work, the next phase of exercise is formatted to strengthen weak muscles.

Muscles that typically need strengthening:

Weak back of shoulders (the posterior deltoids)
Weak shoulder girdle (the external rotator-cuff muscles)
Weak upper back (the rhomboids)
Weak mid back (the latissimus dorsi)
Weak lower back (the erector spinae)
Weak front torso (the abdominal core)
Weak back of upper arms (the triceps)
Weak inner thighs (the vastus medialis)
Weak shin muscles (the tibialis anterior)

Although there are certain muscles that grow weak with inactivity, our bodies have muscle pairings that work in concert with each other. This means that when one muscle becomes stronger, the opposing muscle needs to become relationally stronger as well; this prevents injury and continues to promote good postural alignment. Because of this, it is preferable to pair the exercises to insure balance between opposing muscle groups.

The F.I.T. Prescription

Frequency: Train for strength with a forty-eight-hour rest between sessions to eliminate overtaxing the muscles.

Intensity: Using light resistance, perform one set of twelve to fifteen repetitions per muscle group, as tolerated. To avoid DOMS, eliminate *all* overhead and "holding" exercises; avoid muscle resistance on the eccentric "down phase" of each repetition; alternate sides to give the muscles more rest between repetitions.

Time: A strength training routine will typically take twenty to twenty-five minutes per session.

Progression Step 5—Aerobic Endurance Training

Once the body has established good breathing patterns, has good postural stability, and the muscles are both flexible and strong, it is well prepared to begin endurance training.

As mentioned earlier, there are many forms of aerobic endurance workouts proven well suited to those with FM. We recommend a noncompetitive environment when starting aerobic training. An excellent workout DVD is available on www.myalgia.com with gentle aerobic work that is perfect for those starting this form of exercise. Exercises that are realistic and provide symptom relief in FM enhance the probability of continued activity, in part by bolstering self-efficacy.[22,23]

Although water-based workouts are wonderful when beginning endurance work, be aware they do not provide the slight contact impact needed to increase bone density. It is wise to progress to a land-based, standing endurance workout as soon as possible to help strengthen bones, regain balance, and help prevent osteoporosis.

After six to twelve months of endurance workouts, the participant with FM may find they are able to mainstream into some general fitness programs. Keeping in mind the exercise modalities to avoid, as mentioned in this article, will make all the difference at this point. For instance, overhead machines at the local gym would still not be advisable and the circuit-style programs seen in some popular women's-only gyms involve the type of repetition overload to avoid because of muscle microtrauma.

Those with FM have had success on elliptical trainers, recumbent stationary bikes, and in fitness programs that minimize eccentric work. At this point, a fitness leader or personal trainer would be useful to help design specific exercise instruction. A well-informed fitness professional can tailor exercises to minimize time spent in eccentric contraction, avoid FM tender points, reduce repetitive motion and avoid overhead strength training. Trainers who wish to receive up-to-date, research-based information on exercise precautions for FM clients can visit the following Web site: www.myalgiateam.com.

The F.I.T. Prescription

Frequency: Allow a day off between endurance workouts to recover fully and eliminate DOMS.

Intensity: Avoid *all* overhead movements; alternate movement, change the pace, or break early from overly repetitious patterns.

Time: Begin with ten- to fifteen-minute sessions, increasing by five minutes every four weeks. Remember: Workouts lasting longer than thirty minutes add little benefit, but greatly increase the likelihood of DOMS in those with FM. In the very beginning, it is reasonable to take time between aerobic activities by exercising in three five-minute bouts, spread throughout the day. However, the long-term goal remains one twenty + minute period of aerobic endurance exercise three to four times per week.

SAMPLE TRAINING TABLE

See Table 12.1 for an exercise prescription example, which we have found effective in our FM exercise center.

Key Points:

- Cold or heat can trigger an FM flare.
- If exercising outdoors, dress in layers and wear sunscreen, even in the winter.
- Keep a water bottle handy and keep hydrated.
- Those with arthritis, osteoporosis, tendonitis, bursitis, plantar fasciitis, or low back pain need to move at a slower pace and may want to exercise in a warm therapeutic pool or a chair.
- Protect painful joints with ace wraps, stabilizers or bands.
- A warm shower or hot tub can help reduce post exercise pain.
- Plan rewards to keep motivated.
- Find an exercise pal who understands FM and will be gently encouraging.

Table 12.1
Exercise Prescription Example

Sample Traning Chart								
Week	Time	B	P	FT	ST	WU	ES	CD
1–2	10 to 15 minutes	√	√					
3–8	25 to 30 minutes	√	√	½√		√		
9–12	30 to 45 minutes	√	√	√		√		
13–16	45 minutes to 1 hour	√	√	√	½√	√		
17–20	1 hour		√	√	√	√	½√	√
21–24	1 hour		√	√	√	√	√*	√

B = Breath work   WU = Endurance Warm-Up
P = Postural Alignment   ES = Endurance Session
FT = Flexibility Training   EC = Endurance Cool-Down
ST = Strength Training   *or as tolerated
Source: © JH Hoffman and KD Jones 2007. Courtesy of Kim Jones.

Modifications for Activities of Daily Living

- Take shorter steps when walking downhill to minimize eccentric muscle work.
- Avoid carrying a heavy shoulder bag. This protects upper torso tender points.
- When attending movies or theater venues, arrive early or purchase center seating rather than sitting to the far right or left. This helps avoid side neck strain.
- Always use handrails, and use canes as needed, to help avoid falls.
- Take breaks often when reaching overhead repeatedly.
- Purchase a grabber for reaching objects on high shelves.
- Change positions frequently whenever stationary to avoid muscle tension buildup.
- Use a telephone headset and other ergonomic aids to minimize overuse syndromes or unnatural body positions.

In summary, exercise is safe and effective in FM when prescribed at the proper frequency, intensity, and type. Exercise will improve physical fitness/function and symptoms, especially fatigue, stiffness and sleep problems for this special population.

REFERENCES

1. Jones KD, Ross RL, Adams DG, Bennett RM. "Fibromyalgia: A rational guide for management in primary care." *Clinican Reviews* 16 (2006): 3–13.

2. Wolfe F, Smythe HA, Yunus MB, Bennett RM, Bombardier C, Goldenberg DL, Tugwell P, Campbell SM, Abeles M, Clark P. "The American College of Rheumatology 1990 Criteria for the Classification of Fibromyalgia. Report of the Multicenter Criteria Committee." *Arthritis Rheum* 33 (1990): 160–172.

3. Bennett RM, Jones KD, Turk DC, Russell IJ, Matallana L. "An internet survey of 2,596 people with fibromyalgia." *BioMed Central Rheumatology* 8 (2007): 1–11.

4. Penrod JR, Bernatsky S, Adam V, Baron M, Dayan N, Dobkin PL. "Health services costs and their determinants in women with fibromyalgia." *J Rheumatol* 31 (2004): 1391–1398.

5. White KP, Speechley M, Harth M, Ostbye T. "The London Fibromyalgia Epidemiology Study: Direct health care costs of fibromyalgia syndrome in London, Canada." *J Rheumatol* 26 (1999): 885–889.

6. Moldofsky H, Scarisbrick P, England R, Smythe H. "Musculosketal symptoms and non-REM sleep disturbance in patients with 'fibrositis syndrome' and healthy subjects." *Psychosom Med* 37 (1975): 341–351.

7. Moldofsky H, Scarisbrick P. "Induction of neurasthenic musculoskeletal pain syndrome by selective sleep stage deprivation." *Psychosom Med* 38 (1976): 35–44.

8. McCain GA, Bell DA, Mai FM, Halliday PD. "A controlled study of the effects of a supervised cardiovascular fitness training program on the manifestations of primary fibromyalgia." *Arthritis Rheum* 31 (1988): 1135–1141.

9. Jones KD, Adams D, Winters-Stone K, Burckhardt CS. "A comprehensive review of 46 exercise treatment studies in fibromyalgia (1988–2005)." *Health Qual Life Outcomes* 4 (2006): 67.

10. Jones KD, Clark SR, Bennett RM. "Prescribing exercise for people with fibromyalgia." *AACN Clin Issues* 13 (2002): 277–293.

11. Jones KD, Adams DG. "How to diagnose and treat fibromyalgia." *Arthritis Practitioner* 1 (2005): 14–20.

12. Jones KD, Burckhardt CS, Perrin NA, Hanson G, Deodhar AA, Bennett RM. "Growth hormone response to acute exercise normalizes with long-term pyridostigmine but does not change IGF-1." *J Rheumatol* (2007): In press.

13. Staud R. "Biology and therapy of fibromyalgia: pain in fibromyalgia syndrome." *Arthritis Res Ther* 8 (2006): 208.

14. Bennett RM. "Rational management of fibromyalgia." *Rheum Dis Clin North Am* 28 (2002): xiii–xixv.

15. Jones KD, Horak FB, Winters K, Bennett RM. "Fibromyalgia impairs balance compared to age and gender matched controls [abstract]." *Arthritis & Rheumatism* 59 (2005): S81.

16. Pierrynowski MR, Tiidus PM, Galea V. "Women with fibromyalgia walk with an altered muscle synergy." *Gait Posture* 22 (2005): 210–218.

17. Bigelow SL. *Fibromyalgia: Simple Relief through Movement.* 1st ed. (New York: Wiley, 2000).

18. Turk DC, Winter F. *The Pain Survival Guide: How to Reclaim Your Life.* 1st ed. (Washington, DC: American Psychological Association, 2006).

19. Bennett RM. "The contribution of muscle to the generation of fibromyalgia symptomatology." *J Musculoskeletal Pain* 4(1/2) (1996): 35–59.

20. Clark SR, Jones KD, Burckhardt CS, Bennett R. "Exercise for patients with fibromyalgia: risks versus benefits." *Curr Rheumatol Rep* 3 (2001): 135–146.

21. Farhi D. *The Breathing Book: Good Health and Vitality through Essential Breath Work.* 1st ed. (New York: Henry Holt & Co, 2007).

22. Jones KD, Burckhardt CS, Clark SR, Bennett RM, Potempa KM. "A randomized controlled trial of muscle strengthening versus flexibility training in fibromyalgia." *J Rheumatol* 29 (2002): 1041–1048.

23. Jones KD, Burckhardt CS, Bennett JA. "Motivational interviewing may encourage exercise in persons with fibromyalgia by enhancing self efficacy." *Arthritis Rheum* 51 (2004): 864–867.

13

EXERCISE AND CANCER

Kathleen Y. Wolin

It is estimated that nearly 1.5 million new cases of cancer will be diagnosed in 2007 and there are nearly 11 million survivors in the United States.[1] Of the individuals diagnosed with cancer, 65 percent live five or more years. It is estimated that one-third of the cancer deaths in the United States each year are due to nutrition and physical activity factors, including excess weight. This chapter outlines the evidence that a physically active lifestyle can prevent cancer and then turns to what benefits physical activity might have for individuals undergoing treatment for cancer and cancer survivors.

PREVENTION

History

In 1922, Dr. Thomas Cherry undertook the first study of the relationship between physical activity and cancer prevention.[2] Dr. Cherry studied cancer rates across cities of comparable size in which the predominant occupations involved light or heavy work. Dr. Cherry found that people in cities with predominantly heavy labor professions had lower rates of cancer. Since then hundreds of studies have examined the association between physical activity and the occurrence of cancer. In 1994, the U.S. Surgeon General concluded that a lack of physical activity increases the risk of colon cancer and may increase the risk of breast cancer.[3] In 2002, the International Agency for Research on Cancer issued a report that stated evidence existed to show that physical activity protects against breast and colon cancer.[4] Other researchers have reached similar conclusions for breast and colon cancer and have found suggestive, but less conclusive, evidence for a decreased risk of endometrial, prostate, and lung cancers.[5,6]

Methods Used to Study Physical Activity in Cancer Prevention

Types of Studies

Cancer prevention studies typically appear in one of two forms, which are case control and cohort studies. Case control studies generally enroll individuals with recently diagnosed cancer and equally matched cancer-free subjects (controls). Both sets of individuals then complete questionnaires about their lifestyle, behavior, and environment at a designated period in the past (e.g., one year ago). In cohort studies, a large sample of disease-free individuals is enrolled in the study at one time. These individuals all complete the same questionnaire about their lifestyle, behavior, and environment. Questions can refer to any current or past time period. The cohort is then followed over time for the development of cancer. Assuming that both types of studies are well conducted, usually more weight is given to the results of cohort studies, which are subject to fewer biases (e.g., bias in the recall of prediagnosis behaviors).

Measuring Physical Activity

Research studies have predominantly measured physical activity in two ways: by occupation and by leisure-time activities. Typically, household and transportation-related physical activities have not been included in studies of cancer. For many jobs, occupational activity may be relatively constant from week to week and year to year whereas leisure-time activity is more likely to change daily, weekly, and seasonally. It is well known that, particularly in the United States, job-related energy expenditure has been declining for most population segments. As such, more recent studies of physical activity and cancer prevention have typically focused on leisure-time physical activity with a few studies measuring both occupational and leisure activity.

Leisure-time Physical Activity Measures

To date, most large studies of the association between physical activity and cancer have measured physical activity using questionnaires. A typical questionnaire might ask participants to report how frequently and for what duration in the past week he or she participated in each of a set of activities. Such a list may include walking, running, cycling, tennis, golf, and yoga. Questionnaires often reference current physical activity, but some also inquire about physical activity at a specific point in the past (e.g., puberty, age 20, one year ago, ten years ago). The validity of these questionnaires is quite variable.[4,7]

Because of the challenges associated with measuring physical activity using questionnaires (relying on participants' recollections), there is increasing interest in using more objective measures including pedometers and accelerometers. Unfortunately, these devices have become popular in medical studies only in the last decade or so. Frequently, their cost is prohibitive (accelerometers typically cost over $400 each) in the large studies necessary to study cancer outcomes. In addition, because cancer is a disease that takes many years or even decades to develop, giving a cohort of individuals pedometers today in a prospective study would not provide data about the association with cancer outcomes for many years. In retrospective studies, the physical activity of interest occurs before the diagnosis and thus, can only be measured via recall on a self-report instrument. Thus, for the time being, cancer prevention studies are limited to questionnaire measures of physical activity with its associated challenges.

Colon Cancer

Numerous studies have illustrated a relationship between physical activity and colon cancer. As previously stated, a number of agencies and researchers have found convincing evidence for this relationship. These agencies have, in fact, given the available evidence the highest scientific weight given in studies of cancer causes or protective factors.[4,8,9] Higher levels of physical activity are related to lower rates of colon.

Over thirty case-control studies have been published and most found an inverse relation between both occupational and leisure-time physical activity and colon cancer risk among men and women.

While the first cohort study of physical activity and colon cancer failed to show any protective benefit,[10] most cohort studies show a reduction in risk similar to that observed in the case-control studies. That is, higher activity in adulthood is related to a reduced risk of colon cancer. In some studies, colon and rectal cancers are examined together (i.e., "colorectal cancer"). However, when examined separately, an inverse association between physical activity and rectal cancer is generally not seen whereas an association for colon cancer and physical activity is apparent.

The Harvard Alumni Study, a cohort of Harvard College graduates who matriculated between 1916 and 1950, examined leisure-time physical activity. In that cohort, Lee and colleagues observed a strong inverse association among men who were physically active both in the 1960s and seventeen years later.[11] Men expending more than 2,500 kcal per week in leisure physical activity had a 50 percent reduction in risk of colon cancer compared with those expending less than 1,000 kcal per week. This is roughly the difference between brisk walking for thirty minutes a day and brisk walking for eighty minutes a day.

When occupation was used to categorize activity in a study of Swedish men, those with higher physical activity had a lower risk of colon cancer.[12] In that study the greatest risk reduction was found when classifying men using occupation and leisure physical activity combined. Men in the highest total physical activity group had a 70 percent reduction in risk compared with men who were inactive at work and engaged in little leisure-time activity. Thus, individuals who are physically active in all aspects of their life may have the lowest risk of colon cancer.

Overall, cohort studies conducted in a variety of countries support a dose-response relation across increasing physical activity levels: higher physical activity levels are related to lower levels of colon cancer risk. Those in the highest physical activity category have approximately a 40–50 percent reduction in risk of colon cancer compared to the least physically active category.[13]

Unfortunately, despite the consistent associations seen across study designs, study populations, and physical activity measures, much remains unknown.

What Type of Physical Activities Should I Do?

We don't know if certain types of activity are more beneficial than others. For example, is swimming better than jogging? Emerging research suggests that protective benefit can be obtained by moderate intensity physical activities like walking, but we don't know if a particular type of activity of a similar intensity is better than another.

Moderate Intensity Physical Activity

Moderate intensity physical activity is defined as activity in which a person should experience some increase in breathing or heart rate. Examples of common moderate intensity physical activities include brisk walking, dancing, mowing the lawn (with a motorized pushmower), swimming, or cycling on level terrain.

Do I Need to Have Been Active My Whole Life?

Three studies that address physical activity during early adulthood show no relation to colon cancer risk.[10,14,15] These data suggest that physical activity later in life may be particularly important. Evidence from the Harvard Alumni Study may also support this. Men who had increased their level of activity during follow-up of the cohort had a suggestion of lower risk of colon cancer during subsequent follow-up,[11] but in a later analysis of the data with longer follow-up, no effect was found.[16] In sum, it seems that individuals who were not active in early adulthood can still reduce their risk by becoming physically active later in life.

Are People Who Are Physically Active Just Healthier?

Indeed, healthy lifestyle behaviors do cluster together. In a detailed analysis of the Health Professionals Follow-up Study, a cohort of some 50,000 men followed to study relations between diet and chronic diseases, Giovannucci et al. showed that individuals with higher physical activity were more likely to use multivitamins and had higher intakes of fiber. They also had a lower intake of saturated fat, a lower prevalence of cigarette smoking, and lower body mass index.[17] Many of the studies that report an association between physical activity and colon cancer have controlled for other lifestyle factors (e.g., body weight, alcohol intake, diet) that may be associated with physical activity. The inverse relation between physical activity and colon cancer is not materially altered when investigators have controlled for these other lifestyle factors. Thus, we can conclude that physical activity is not merely a marker of healthier lifestyle, but exerts an independent protective effect.

What Is the Biological Link between Physical Activity and Colon Cancer?

Several biologic mechanisms have been proposed though no conclusive data exists. Insulin may play a role in mediating the association between physical activity and colon cancer as insulin sensitivity improves with exercise. Insulin also promotes the growth of colon mucosal cells in laboratory and animal studies. Thus, it is possible that activity exerts its protective effect through reduced insulin levels. Physical activity also induces changes in other cellular growth factors. Finally, some have suggested that physical activity decreases intestinal transit time, reducing the exposure of the colon to potential carcinogens.

Despite these questions, a large body of evidence supports the conclusion that higher levels of physical activity result in a lower risk of colon cancer.

Breast Cancer

In addition to concluding that evidence exists for a protective effect of physical activity on colon cancer, convincing evidence shows that physical activity reduces the risk of breast cancer. Risk reduction ranges from 10 to 70 percent, with average decrease in risk of 20–40 percent, when comparing the most and least physically active women.[4,18] Like colon cancer, this risk reduction is seen across physical activity domains (e.g., leisure, occupational, total [which is generally comprised of leisure, occupational, household/yard/domestic, and transportation physical activity combined]).

The benefits of physical activity are seen in both pre and postmenopausal women. Evidence suggests physical activity may be particularly important in decreasing risk of postmenopausal breast cancer because of the role of physical activity in controlling weight gain, a key modifiable risk factor for postmenopausal breast cancer.

It is believed that physical activity reduces breast cancer risk by reducing hormone levels, though the exact mechanisms likely vary with age. In young girls, physical activity delays menarche (the onset of menstruation), which is known to reduce risk of breast cancer. Once menstruation has been established, physically active women may be exposed to fewer hormones as they are more likely to experience anovulatory and irregular menstrual cycles. In postmenopausal women, physical activity influences fat stores, which are the body's primary source of estrogen.

Prostate Cancer

Evidence is less strong, though generally considered probable, that physical activity protects against prostate cancer.[8] In the Health Professional's

Follow-up Study, Giovannucci et al. found that men who participated in the most physical activity had a 30 percent lower risk of prostate cancer than those who were least physically active.[19] When comparing the cardiovascular fitness of men in a separate cohort, Oliveria and colleagues reported those who were most fit had a 70 percent lower risk of prostate cancer than men who were least fit.[20] Generally, prostate cancer risk reductions of 20–50 percent are found when comparing the most and least physically active men. Similar to colon and breast cancers, both leisure and occupational physical activity have shown a protective benefit for prostate cancer.

Unfortunately, the biology of prostate cancer is poorly understood, limiting our ability to understand the mechanisms by which physical activity may reduce risk. In general, it is known that physical activity enhances immune functioning and while strenuous exercise has been shown to alter hormone levels, its influence on testosterone levels is less clear. Physically active men have been found to have lower serum testosterone levels, but most studies indicate that the association between physical activity and testosterone level is mediated by body composition.

Endometrial Cancer

Similar to prostate cancer, probable or possible[8] evidence exists that physical activity reduces the risk of endometrial cancer. Generally, risk reductions of 20–40 percent are reported for both occupational and leisure physical activity. Similar to breast cancer, pathways related to decreased hormone circulation and decreased fat mass are believed to drive the associations.

Lung Cancer

Of the few studies evaluating the association between physical activity and lung cancer, most have found an inverse relationship. Risk reductions were moderate in size. However, given the limited amount of data available, the association can only be classified as possible.

Conclusion

Generally speaking, research is limited on the type, intensity, duration, and long-term patterns of physical activity necessary to reduce risk of cancer. Greater protection may come from participation in more vigorous physical activities (e.g., jogging, bicycling uphill, high impact aerobics or aerobic dance, lawn mowing with a nonmotorized pushmower). It has been suggested that long-term involvement in physical activity is important in reducing cancer risk, but the evidence varies by cancer site. There is substantial evidence that physical activity is associated with reduced risk of several cancers, most notably colon and breast cancer. There is less consistent evidence of an association with several other cancers. While the exact amount and type of physical activity necessary for protection is not precisely known, participation in thirty minutes of physical activity of at least moderate intensity on most days of the week appears sufficient to reduce risk of several cancers.

TREATMENT AND SURVIVAL

As with any population, but particularly for those with chronic illnesses like cancer, one should consult your physician before starting any exercise program. Caution should be employed when selecting an exercise program, but many patients experience benefits of engaging in exercise before, during, and after treatment. For older individuals or those with bone disease or other impairments, particular attention should be paid to maintaining balance and reducing the risk of falls during physical activity. Survivors with anemia should consult a physician before beginning a physical activity program. Individuals with compromised immune function may want to avoid public exercise facilities. Physicians and patients can refer to the detailed summary of the latest evidence provided by the American Cancer Society in Doyle C, et al. Nutrition and Physical Activity During and After Cancer Treatment: An American Cancer Society Guide for Informed Choices. *CA Cancer J Clin* 2006; 56:323–353.

History

Compared to the wealth of data on the benefits of physical activity for cancer prevention, relatively little data is available on the effects of physical activity following cancer diagnosis. Most of the studies in the area of physical activity among cancer patients and survivors have focused on intermediate outcomes including depression, fatigue, functioning, and quality of life. Only a handful of studies have examined the effect of physical activity after diagnosis on survival. The majority of the research on physical activity following cancer diagnosis has occurred in breast cancer patients.

Historically, cancer patients were discouraged from being physically active during treatment. However, a sedentary lifestyle increases risks for other adverse health outcomes and may limit activities of daily living. It is perhaps not surprising then that when researchers asked cancer survivors many reported being regularly physically active,[21] though generally at levels that are lower than prediagnosis.

Breast Cancer

Data is promising for the beneficial effects of physical activity during treatment for breast cancer. Several studies have compared quality of life before and after an exercise intervention and found significant improvements.[22,23] Physical activity programs, not surprisingly, also frequently lead to improvements in strength and fitness.[22,23]

Increasingly, researchers are enrolling women in randomized intervention trials. Much like studies of medications, well-conducted randomized trials are considered the gold standard in research. Participants in these trials are randomly assigned to one of two (or more) types of treatments: an exercise intervention or control. Data from randomized trials with a control group are generally given more weight when reviewing evidence than those studies that compare participants' own values before and after an intervention.

Among women on adjuvant treatment, Campbell and colleagues found a twelve-week program of aerobic and resistance exercise leads to improvements in fitness and functional status as compared to receiving usual care.[24] Similarly, Courneya and colleagues found a fifteen-week aerobic exercise intervention leads to improvements in fitness, quality of life, strength, and well-being as well as a decrease in fatigue as compared to a no exercise control group.[25] Additional studies have had similar findings.[26-28] While many trials have studied the effects of aerobic exercise, others have found significant benefits for nonaerobic exercise. For example, Schmitz and colleagues reported significant physiologic changes following a strength training intervention.[29] Other randomized studies have not found a significant effect for physiologic or psychological measures when comparing intervention and control groups but have found significant changes within the intervention group from baseline to study end.[30-33] While these results are less convincing, combined with the significant intervention effects seen elsewhere, the body of evidence does seem promising for many beneficial effects of exercise programs in women with breast cancer.

More recently researchers have tapped the large observational studies used to look at cancer prevention to understand the role of exercise in survival. Holmes and colleagues, using the Nurses' Health Study cohort, found that compared to the least active women, women who were the most active after diagnosis of breast cancer had nearly a 50 percent lower risk of death.

Colorectal Cancer

In the one study of colorectal cancer patients on adjuvant therapy, Courneya and colleagues have found that sixteen weeks of cardiovascular and flexibility exercises had no significant effect on quality of life or fitness as compared with a no exercise control group.[34] However, over half of the control group exercised, which would dilute the effect of the intervention.

Large observational studies have found that physical activity after diagnosis of colon cancer improves overall, recurrence-free, and disease-free survival.[35,36] The influence of prediagnosis physical activity is less clear, with one study showing a protective benefit[37] and another finding no association.[35]

Mixed Diagnosis

In studies of multiple cancer diagnoses, some[38–40] researchers have not found a significant change in quality of life after an exercise intervention. Results are also equivocal for the effect of physical activity on cancer-related fatigue.[41,42] As with single diagnosis studies, physical activity programs lead to improvements in strength and fitness.[38,40,41,43–45]

Possible Benefits of Regular Exercise during Cancer Treatment

- Maintain or improvement physical abilities
- Improvement balance, reducing risk of falls and fractures
- Prevention of muscle wasting caused by inactivity
- Reduced risk of heart disease
- Prevention of osteoporosis
- Imporved blood flow to legs and reduced risk of blood clots
- Less dependence on others to do normal activities of daily living
- Improved self-esteem
- Reduced anxiety and depression
- Decreased nausea
- Increased ability to maintain social contact
- Reduced symtoms of fatigue
- Better ability to control weight
- Improved quality of life

Source: Reprinted with permission of the American Cancer Society, Inc. from www. cancer.org. All right reserved.

Conclusions

Exercise in cancer survivors may lead to positive psychological and physiological changes including better quality of life and physical functioning. However, additional studies are needed as drawing conclusions from such a diverse set of studies is challenging. The interventions studied have ranged from two to twenty weeks and included aerobic, resistance, and flexibility, both singularly and jointly. The patient populations have included individuals on active treatment, adjuvant treatment (i.e., treatment given to boost the effectiveness of the primary treatment), and post treatment. Thus, it has been difficult for clinicians and patients to decide the best course of action. In many cases, recommendations are based on research in healthy populations. For example, we know that in adults without cancer, resistance training can offset aging-related bone loss. Thus, clinicians often recommend exercise to cancer patients on hormone therapies to offset the bone loss associated with the treatment. In general, exercise appears safe for cancer patients and survivors and research has found positive benefits of physical activity in cancer patients and survivors.

REFERENCES

1. American Cancer Society. *Cancer Facts and Figures 2007* (Atlanta, GA: American Cancer Society, 2007).

2. Cherry T. "A theory of cancer." *Med J Australia* 1(1922): 425–438.

3. U.S. Department of Health and Human Services. *Physical activity and health: A report of the Surgeon General* (Atlanta, GA: U.S. Department of Health and Human Services, Centers for Disease Control and Prevention, National Center for Chronic Disease Prevention and Health Promotion, 1996).

4. International Agency for Research on Cancer WHO. *IARC Handbooks of Cancer Prevention: Weight Control and Physical Activity*, Volume 6 (Lyon, France: International Agency for Research on Cancer, 2002).

5. McTiernan A, Ulrich C, Slate S, Potter J. "Physical activity and cancer etiology: Associations and mechanisms." *Cancer Causes Control* 9 (1998): 487–509.

6. Marrett LD, Theis B, Ashbury FD. "Workshop report: Physical activity and cancer prevention." *Chronic Dis Can* 21 (2004): 143–149.

7. Jacobs DR, Jr., Ainsworth BE, Hartman TJ, Leon AS. "A simultaneous evaluation of 10 commonly used physical activity questionnaires." *Med Sci Sports Exerc* 25 (1993): 81–91.

8. Friedenreich CM. "Physical activity and cancer prevention: From observational to intervention research." *Cancer Epidemiol Biomarkers Prev* 10 (2001): 287–301.

9. Byers T, Nestle M, McTiernan A, et al. "American Cancer Society guidelines on nutrition and physical activity for cancer prevention: Reducing the risk of cancer with healthy food choices and physical activity." *CA Cancer J Clin* 52 (2002): 92–119.

10. King G, Polednak AP, Bendel R, Hovey D. "Cigarette smoking among native and foreign-born African Americans." *Ann Epidemiol* May 9 (1999): 236–244.

11. Lee IM, Paffenbarger RS, Jr., Hsieh C. "Physical activity and risk of developing colorectal cancer among college alumni." *J Natl Cancer Inst* 83(1991): 1324–1329.

12. Gerhardsson M, Floderus B, Norell SE. "Physical activity and colon cancer risk." *Int J Epidemiol* 17 (1988): 743–746.

13. Colditz GA, Cannuscio CC, Frazier AL. "Physical activity and reduced risk of colon cancer: Implications for prevention." *Cancer Causes Control* 8 (1997): 649–667.

14. Paffenbarger RS, Jr., Hyde RT, Wing AL. "Physical activity and incidence of cancer in diverse populations: a preliminary report." *Am J Clin Nutr* 45 (1987): 312–317.

15. Marcus PM, Newcomb PA, Storer BE. "Early adulthood physical activity and colon cancer risk among Wisconsin women." *Cancer Epidemiol Biomarkers Prev* 3 (1994): 641–644.

16. Lee IM, Paffenbarger RS, Jr. "Physical activity and its relation to cancer risk: A prospective study of college alumni." *Med Sci Sports Exerc* 26 (1994): 831–837.

17. Giovannucci E, Ascherio A, Rimm EB, Colditz GA, Stampfer MJ, Willett WC. "Physical activity, obesity, and risk for colon cancer and adenoma in men." *Ann Intern Med* 122 (1995): 327–334.

18. Brinton LA, Bernstein L, Colditz GA. "Summary of the workshop: Workshop on Physical Activity and Breast Cancer, November 13–14, 1997." *Cancer* 83 (1998): 595–599.

19. Giovannucci E, Leitzmann M, Spiegelman D, et al. "A prospective study of physical activity and prostate cancer in male health professionals." *Cancer Res* 58 (1998): 5117–5122.

20. Oliveria SA, Kohl HW, 3rd, Trichopoulos D, Blair SN. "The association between cardiorespiratory fitness and prostate cancer." *Med Sci Sports Exerc* 28 (1996): 97–104.

21. Demark-Wahnefried W, Peterson B, McBride C, Lipkus I, Clipp E. "Current health behaviors and readiness to pursue life-style changes among men and women diagnosed with early stage prostate and breast carcinomas." *Cancer* 88 (2000): 674–684.

22. Goodwin P, Esplen MJ, Butler K, et al." Multidisciplinary weight management in locoregional breast cancer: results of a phase II study." *Breast Cancer Res Treat* 48 (1998): 53–64.

23. Kolden GG, Strauman TJ, Ward A, et al. "A pilot study of group exercise training (GET) for women with primary breast cancer: feasibility and health benefits." *Psychooncology* 11 (2002): 447–456.

24. Campbell A, Mutrie N, White F, McGuire F, Kearney N. "A pilot study of a supervised group exercise programme as a rehabilitation treatment for women with breast cancer receiving adjuvant treatment." *Eur J Oncol Nurs* 9 (2005): 56–63.

25. Courneya KS, Mackey JR, Bell GJ, Jones LW, Field CJ, Fairey AS. "Randomized controlled trial of exercise training in postmenopausal breast cancer survivors: cardiopulmonary and quality of life outcomes." *J Clin Oncol* 21 (2003): 1660–1668.

26. Schwartz AL, Mori M, Gao R, Nail LM, King ME. "Exercise reduces daily fatigue in women with breast cancer receiving chemotherapy." *Med Sci Sports Exerc* 33 (2001): 718–723.

27. Winningham ML, MacVicar MG, Bondoc M, Anderson JI, Minton JP. "Effect of aerobic exercise on body weight and composition in patients with breast cancer on adjuvant chemotherapy." *Oncol Nurs Forum* 16 (1989): 683–689.

28. Segar ML, Katch VL, Roth RS, et al. "The effect of aerobic exercise on self-esteem and depressive and anxiety symptoms among breast cancer survivors." *Oncol Nurs Forum* 25 (1998): 107–113.

29. Schmitz KH, Holtzman J, Courneya KS, Masse LC, Duval S, Kane R. "Controlled physical activity trials in cancer survivors: a systematic review and meta-analysis." *Cancer Epidemiol Biomarkers Prev* 14 (2005): 1588–1595.

30. Pinto BM, Clark MM, Maruyama NC, Feder SI. "Psychological and fitness changes associated with exercise participation among women with breast cancer." *Psychooncology* 12 (2003): 118–126.

31. Pinto BM, Frierson GM, Rabin C, Trunzo JJ, Marcus BH. "Home-based physical activity intervention for breast cancer patients." *J Clin Oncol* 23 (2005): 3577–3587.

32. Mock V, Frangakis C, Davidson NE, et al. "Exercise manages fatigue during breast cancer treatment: a randomized controlled trial." *Psychooncology* 14 (2005): 464–477.

33. McKenzie DC, Kalda AL. "Effect of upper extremity exercise on secondary lymphedema in breast cancer patients: a pilot study." *J Clin Oncol* 21 (2003): 463–466.

34. Courneya KS, Friedenreich CM, Quinney HA, Fields AL, Jones LW, Fairey AS. "A randomized trial of exercise and quality of life in colorectal cancer survivors." *Eur J Cancer Care* 12 (2003): 347–357.

35. Meyerhardt JA, Giovannucci EL, Holmes MD, et al. "Physical activity and survival after colorectal cancer diagnosis." *J Clin Oncol* 24 (2006): 3527–3534.

36. Meyerhardt JA, Heseltine D, Niedzwiecki D, et al. "Impact of physical activity on cancer recurrence and survival in patients with stage III colon cancer: findings from CALGB 89803." *J Clin Oncol* 24 (2006): 3535–3541.

37. Haydon AM, Macinnis RJ, English DR, Giles GG. "Effect of physical activity and body size on survival after diagnosis with colorectal cancer." *Gut* 55 (2006): 62–67.

38. Burnham TR, Wilcox A. "Effects of exercise on physiological and psychological variables in cancer survivors." *Med Sci Sports Exer* 34 (2002): 1863–1867.

39. Durak EP, Lilly PC. "The application of exercise and wellness program for cancer patients: A preliminary report." *Journal of Strength and Conditioning Research* 12 (1998): 3–6.

40. Adamsen L, Midtgaard J, Rorth M, et al. "Feasibility, physical capacity, and health benefits of a multidimensional exercise program for cancer patients undergoing chemotherapy." *Support Care Cancer* 11 (2003): 707–716.

41. Dimeo F, Rumberger BG, Keul J. "Aerobic exercise as therapy for cancer fatigue." *Med Sci Sports Exerc* 30 (1998): 475–478.

42. Dimeo FC, Stieglitz RD, Novelli-Fischer U, Fetscher S, Keul J. "Effects of physical activity on the fatigue and psychologic status of cancer patients during chemotherapy." *Cancer* 85 (1999): 2273–2277.

43. Dimeo FC, Tilmann MH, Bertz H, Kanz L, Mertelsmann R, Keul J. "Aerobic exercise in the rehabilitation of cancer patients after high dose chemotherapy and autologous peripheral stem cell transplantation." *Cancer* 79 (1997): 1717–1722.

44. Hayes S, Davies PS, Parker T, Bashford J. "Total energy expenditure and body composition changes following peripheral blood stem cell transplantation and participation in an exercise programme." *Bone Marrow Transplant* 31 (2003): 331–338.

45. Durak EP, Lilly PC, Hackworth JL. "Physical and psychosocial responses to exercise in cancer patients: A two year follow-up survey with prostate, leukemia, and general carcinoma." *Journal of Exercise Physiology* 2 (1999): 1–10.

14

EXERCISE AND GASTROINTESTINAL DISORDERS

Gerard Mullin and Ghazaleh Aram

Are you one of the 90 million Americans with a diagnosed digestive condition or one the countless many who have symptoms and are not under the care of a physician? If so, you may be one of the over 50 percent of individuals with diagnosed gastrointestinal disease who use holistic alternatives for self-improvement. There are a number of treatment alternatives that favorably modify digestive illnesses. Diet, supplements, herbal preparations, yoga, meditation, and mind-body interventions have been shown to improve digestive disease outcome. Can exercise positively influence digestive health and mitigate gastrointestinal disease? Certainly exercise is important in promoting health in general and has significant effects on some organ systems such as the heart and blood vessels.

As much as the cardiovascular system is the delivery system for transporting vital nutrients and oxygen to the body's metabolic machinery, the digestive system is the body's refinery, which processes crude ingredients into fuel for the body. Part of the digestive system, the liver, is the body's metabolic power plant with thousands of enzymes and biochemical reactions. Since exercise has been proven to improve blood circulation and its oxygen-carrying capacity along with many changes in metabolism, it seems logical to assume that exercise can influence digestion. There are many perceptions of the health benefits of exercise on digestive health.

In this chapter, we will review the latest research and the impact of exercise on digestive health and disease. One key concept to keep in mind is that the level of intensity in exercise can impact on the gastrointestinal system in different ways. More isn't necessarily better!

EXERCISE IN SPECIFIC GI CONDITIONS

Gastroesophageal Reflux Disease

Gastroesophageal reflux disease (GERD) is a condition that is characterized by the regurgitation of the stomach's digestive contents into the conduit of the digestive system, the esophagus. It has been well described that competitive athletes, especially runners, do report increased symptoms of reflux during exercise that limits their training and competition.[1,2] Furthermore, strenuous exercise may cause a gammit of upper gastrointestinal symptoms such as bloating, regurgitation, belching, heartburn, abdominal fullness, and chest pain in up to 45–90 percent of athletes.[3] Cyclists, doing stationary training, produce the least amount of body agitation and have the least amount of reflux. Running on the other hand, an aerobic exercise that involves a high-degree of body movement, has the highest degree of reflux compared to weight training (anaerobic) or biking.[4] Thus, a fasting state is better for running, cycling, and other exercises requiring high levels of body agitation. The cause for these episodes of reflux are thought to be due to relaxation of the esophageal valve that normally keeps contents of the stomach from backing up into the esophagus. These transient lower esophageal sphincter relaxations are worsened after a meal because of abdominal distention, increased abdominal pressure, and air swallowing that occurs during meal consumption. Preliminary studies indicate that acid-reducing agents may prevent and treat acid reflux, however other confirmatory studies are required to know for sure whether acid-reducing agents alters the reflux symptoms of these athletes.[5,6] For the runner or anyone who exercises, the occurrence of chest pain raises serious concerns for the presence of cardiovascular disease. A prompt medical evaluation for an underlying cardiovascular cause is mandatory for chest pain. Once cardiovascular disease is excluded, GERD should be considered as the next possible cause of chest pain, since acid reflux can oftentimes be confused for angina. Therefore, if reflux is a bothersome component in one's training, considerations must be given to switching the mode of exercise (for example changing from running to stationary aerobic exercise) and also fasting state to decrease events of reflux.

Gastric Emptying and Gastric Acid Production

Exercise does stimulate the pumping action of the stomach under conditions of light exercise and can shorten gastric transit,[7] however there are other studies showing no effect.[8] The rate of gastric emptying does not seem to be significantly affected until the point of heavy physical exercise that exceeds 70 percent of maximum oxygen consumption. Electrolyte repletion is very important in the liquid form to rehydrate oneself during moderate to heavy exercise regimens. Athletes should be mindful that heavy physical exertion may delay rehydration efforts. The exact cause of delayed emptying with vigorous exercise is unknown, but it is assumed to be due to the increased stress hormones (catecholamines) that tend to freeze digestive functions in the setting of emergencies. Furthermore, endogenous opioids are released during exercise, which slow intestinal transit much like prescription narcotics. As far as gastric secretion, with light or moderate level of exercise, there is no notable change in acid level in the stomach, however, with intense exercise, gastric acid production is suppressed due to the body's emergency shut off system

Table 14.1
The Effect of Different Parameters on Gastric Emptying

Parameters	Effect on Gastric Emptying
Solute temperature	Warmer fluid consistently delays emptying.
Volume ingested	Gastric emptying rate increases in proportion to the volume ingested. Maximal emptying rate is attained at a volume of 600mL.
$\%Vo_2$ max	Exercise at $\leq 70\%$ Vo_2 max has little effect on gastric emptying, but $>70\%$ Vo_2 max inhibits emptying.
Glucose concentration	Concentration >139mg/dl induces a significant delay in gastric emptying.

Vo_2 max = maximum oxygen consumption.

during fight or flight stressful situations as noted above. In summary, light exercise may enhance while intense exertion impairs gastric movement and function. Submaximal aerobic exercise does not adversely affect gastric transit and should be well tolerated in most healthy athletes. Replacement fluids containing low-osmolality solutions can be given without concerns for impaired delivery or absorption. On the other hand, a marathon runner requires sugar-based solutions with higher caloric intake while running to sustain his or her carbohydrate reserve for continued long-distance running. Given the effects of exertional exercise on gastric transit, greater frequency of smaller quantities of sugar-based drinks should be administered cautiously in order to avoid discomfort. Please refer to Table 14.1 regarding the role of temperature, volume ingested, glucose, and other parameters that are important in gastric emptying.

Peptic Ulcer Disease

It is well known that Helicobacter pylori infections and nonsteroidal antiinflammatory agents are the leading cause of peptic ulcer disease in the world. In general, it is thought that moderate levels of exercise may have beneficial effects on reducing the rates of peptic ulcer disease. One study reported that moderate physical activity was associated with a lower risk of duodenal ulcers in men.[9] Possible mechanisms may include stress reduction, improved sense of well-being, better coping skills, decreased production of stomach acid, and enhanced immune function. Other studies have shown that individuals with occupations requiring high levels of physical activity reported the opposite results but did not control for other lifestyle risks for peptic ulcer disease (i.e., smoking, alcohol, socioeconomic status, etc.).[10]

Inflammatory Bowel Disease (IBD)

Inflammatory bowel disease (IBD) is a chronic relapsing illness characterized by persistent intestinal inflammation, disabling symptoms, higher risk for colorectal cancer, and the need for surgery at times. IBD is associated with loss of bone mass from malabsorption of calcium and vitamin D and/or medications used to treat IBD such as corticosteroids. Exercise and physical activity have been shown to prevent and reverse this loss of bone mass in IBD. Some retrospective studies suggest with regular exercise regimen, there may be a reduction in the relative risk of developing IBD. Individuals having occupations involving physical activity and an open-air environment have a lower incidence of both forms of IBD (ulcerative colitis and Crohn's disease).[11,12] These authors reported that individuals with sedentary occupations and office jobs were at a higher risk for IBD. A subsequent study from Sweden found that individuals who exercised regularly had a significantly lower risk of developing Crohn's Disease.[13] These retrospective studies call for larger scale prospective analyses to validate the protective and preventive role of exercise in IBD. There is also an animal-based study that demonstrated increased intestinal permeability (gut leakiness) after sustained severe exercise in sled dogs.[3] It has not been determined if the above-mentioned factors affect nutrient digestibility. Patients with Crohn's Disease have "leaky guts" (intestinal lumen inflamed and loss of the lumen barrier) that reflect intestinal injury and can be seen in low-blood flow states. Furthermore, a study in dogs showed that during severe exercise nutrient digestibility is impaired.[14] Thus, light to moderate exercise appears to have health benefit, however the impact of severe exercise from limited data may not support this form of physical activity in this population. The section on gastrointestinal bleeding and intestinal injury as a consequence will support this recommendation for the IBD population.

In general, the exact safety of exercise in patients with IBD is unknown, but it is thought that those in remission can tolerate and may benefit from short-term moderate levels of exercise.[15] Physical health, general well-being, quality of life, and perceived stress significantly improve when Crohn's Disease patients undergo a twelve-week exercise program that involves walking three times per week.[16] One possible way that exercise can benefit IBD is through its effects on improving immune homeostasis. Studies looking at the role of immune system have shown that with exercise, certain chemicals may be released in the body that may be protective against the development of inflammatory bowel disease.[17–20]

As mentioned, bone health is an important issue in IBD, especially for Crohn's Disease. Loss of bone density or osteoporosis can be seen in up to 78 percent of patients with IBD.[21] Patients with IBD are more prone to this condition, either due to malabsorption of vitamin D and calcium, or due to the corticosteroids or immunosuppressants that predispose toward thinning of bones. The risk of fractures is 40 percent higher in patients with IBD and it is probably safest to first assess for level of bone disease by bone densitometry and to then consult with a physician for advice about what level of intensity of exercise would be safe and appropriate for each individual.[22] Although it is thought that weight-bearing exercise is the best mode of exercise to prevent bone loss in postmenopausal women, there is no direct data in people with IBD to make the same conclusions. Again, it is best to consult with one's physician in these circumstances to decide what the best exercise regimen would be for each individual with IBD.

In summary, light exercise can promote overall fitness in IBD patients, contribute toward bone health, and support immune function without compromising the underlying disease. Future studies to clarify the types, intensity, and duration of exercise for each IBD subtype along with effects on the immune system would be helpful. Such data would assist physicians to construct individually tailored and carefully monitored physical training programs to improve overall health and well-being.

Constipation and Gastrointestinal Motility

Constipation is a very common problem, especially for those over 65 years of age. Regular physical exercise has been long advocated as a first-line standard of treatment for chronic constipation. It has been well-established that sedentary, bedridden patients are more susceptible to constipation. The general belief is that exercise and physical activity will shorten the gastrointestinal transit time, however, this is not known for certain. Effects of exercise on gastrointestinal motility, such as disruptions of the electrical pacemaker of the gut, the migrating myoelectric complex (MMC),[23,24] and reduced mucosal blood flow have been described.[25] The data from studies analyzing the impact of aerobic exercise on gastrointestinal transit has been inconsistent (see Table 14.2).

In many of these studies, there has been interference from other possible influences such as increased fiber and water in the diet, which facilitate gastrointestinal transit. So far the data available on the role of exercise to improve constipation is inconsistent and unreliable. The presumption is that bowel transit is reduced during heavy exercise due to activation of the body's fight and flight response, but this is not known for certain at this point. In summary, the perception that running consistently improves bowel transit is without merit. Whether light exercise and walking alone improves chronic constipation in otherwise healthy individuals is unclear. Those who are sedentary with chronic constipation can achieve benefit by light to moderate exercise. Overall, the data suggests that exercise provides a benefit without adverse consequences for constipation.

Colorectal Cancer

Colorectal cancer is the third leading cause of cancer incidence and mortality in U.S. men and women. A Western lifestyle, characterized by physical inactivity, a higher caloric intake and the resultant weight gain and obesity plays a major etiologic role. Colorectal cancer is preventable by diet, screening colonoscopy to detect early precancerous lesions, and supplementation with calcium and other agents. Does exercise play a preventive role in the development of colorectal cancer? The data that exercise has a protective effect against

Table 14.2
Impact of Aerobic Exercise on Gastrointestinal Transit

Author, Year	Subjects	Type/ Level of Exercise	Dietary Control	Study Endpoint	Effect on Bowel Transit	Evidence Category
Cammack, 1982	6 healthy young volunteers	6 hours of intermittent bicycling	Standard diet during protocol	Small bowel transit time	No effect	A
Bingham, 1989	14 young, healthy, yet sedentary men and women	9-week running program	Standard diet during protocol	Total bowel transit time	No effect	A
Cordain, 1986	17 young and healthy but untrained men	6-week running program	Dietary question- naire	Total bowel transit time	Significantly reduced	B
Keeling, 1987	12 young active men	Mild treadmill walking	12-hour fast followed by liquid meal	Oro-cecal transit time	Reduced by 20%–25%	B
Oettle, 1991	10 healthy, active, young men and women	3 weeks of moderate exercise	24- hour record of diet	Total bowel transit time	Significantly reduced	B
Coenen, 1991	20 young men	3 days of moderate jogging	Standard diet	Total bowel transit time	No effect	B
Soffer, 1991	8 trained male cyclists	2 days of intense cycling	Standard diet	Oro-cecal transit time	No effect	A
Sesboue, 1995	11 male soccer players and 9 sedentary men	Normal activities	Standard diet guideline not enforced	Large bowel transit time	No difference in two groups	A
Meshkinpur, 1989	23 young, healthy men and women	Light aerobic exercise	Overnight fast then liquid diet	Oro-cecal transit time	Prolonged transit time	A
Van Nieuwen- hoven, 1999	10 well- trained men	High intensity cycling	Standard diet during study	Oro-cecal transit time	No charge	A

Category A = evidence from well-designed controlled clinical trials.
Category B = evidence from cohort or case-controlled studies.

colon cancer is overwhelmingly consistent. However, this data cannot be generalized to rectal cancer per se. The rectum is the last portion of the colon near the anus and cancers of this area have not been shown to be affected by exercise. Therefore, the data that will be discussed in this section mainly applies to colon cancer. The results are striking; nearly all studies have shown a protective role of physical activities on widely varied populations (United States, China, Japan, Hawaii, Western Europe).[26–40] The protective effect of physical exercise is seen across all ethnicities and sexes. The protective effect is less convincing for rectal cancer than for colon cancer.[30–32,38]

The reduction in colon cancer risk is found for increased recreational and occupational activities. Physically active men and women can experience less than half the risk of their sedentary counterparts.[41,42] There has been some discussion that individuals who engage in regular exercise tend to be trim, smoke and drink alcohol less, take aspirin, multivitamins and calcium, and adhere to healthier dietary practices that contribute toward their reduced risk of developing colorectal cancer. Dr. Giovanucci and colleagues investigated whether these other healthy behaviors were really causing the reduction in colon cancers in those who exercise.[32] He prospectively enrolled 47,723 middle-aged to elderly male health professionals to examine whether physical activity independently decreased the risk for colon cancer when controlling for these other healthy behaviors. Their findings indicated that physical activity alone was an independent risk-reducing behavior and that men who undertook the highest levels of activity had the lowest incidence of colon cancer. These men with the highest physical activity had approximately one-half the incidence of developing colon cancer when compared to men with the lowest degree of physical activity. Other studies reproduced their findings as well.[27,28]

Since physical exercise helps to prevent the development of colorectal cancer, how much is needed to achieve a significant health benefit? There are two large studies of note that investigate dose-related responses of exercise on colon cancer rate reduction.[31,42] The Harvard Alumni Study[31] followed 17,148 men for a maximum of twenty-six years. During the study, 225 men developed colon cancer. The men who participated in physical activity equivalent to at least thirty minutes per day, five days per week, had a 50 percent reduction in colon cancer rates compared with men who were sedentary. Physical activity was defined in this study as both the time set aside for daily exercise, as well as other daily physical activities such as climbing stairs. The Nurses Health Study[43] followed more than 67,000 women over six years; 212 women developed colon cancer during the study period. Women who participated in four hours of exercise per week showed a 33 percent risk reduction for colon cancer. Those who exercised more than five hours per week showed a reduction of 46 percent. The physical activity level in the Nurses Health Study was defined as exercise and recreational activity but not ordinary daily activities.

How can exercise help prevent colorectal cancer? What is the latest evidence? The development of colorectal cancer has been long-attributed to the prolonged contact of dietary procarcinogens that are activated by intestinal bacteria and transformed into carcinogens within the intestinal lining. Exercise had been traditionally thought to benefit its cancer protective effect by shortening intestinal transit time (accelerating intestinal movement) and hence, decreasing the time of toxin exposure to the intestinal lining. This theory is not firmly supported by data, since altered intestinal movement have not been consistently shown by a number of researchers.[43–46] Revolutionary theory of colorectal cancer chemoprevention is that exercise strengthens the immune system by promoting the function of many types of immune cells that prevent and fight cancer, including natural killer cells.[47,48] Another possible mechanism is that exercise imparts protection from colorectal cancer by improving insulin responses to meals. Insulin and insulin-like growth factors appear to promote the growth of colorectal cancer in laboratory and animal studies.[28,49–52] Thus, the hyperinsulinism that is associated with obesity, type 2 diabetes, and the metabolic syndrome (syndrome X) may be the means by which these conditions predispose toward the development of colorectal cancer. Finally, exercise is able to ward off unwanted cellular proliferation as well as decreasing some factors such as prostaglandin E2 that is thought to promote colon cell proliferation. This is the biochemical means by which aspirin and nonsteroidal antiinflammatory agents along with Curcumin appear to act in the prevention of colorectal neoplasia.[53–55]

Exercise is becoming an important component of cancer rehabilitation programs. A consistent finding across studies is that patients experience improved physical fitness and reduced fatigue.[56] Exercising during chemotherapy can be challenging. Mustian and colleagues reported on a nationwide population sample of 749 men and women on exercise participation during and within six months after chemotherapy and radiation therapy, the association of exercise with treatment side effects, and the communication between physicians and patients about exercise.[57] Results demonstrated that exercise was associated with less severe side effects during and after treatment. Patients were more likely to continue to exercise if their physician discussed exercise with them. They concluded that cancer patients appear amenable to attempting exercise during and within six months after treatment.

A study that examined the effects of aerobic exercise on physiologic and psychologic function in patients rehabilitating from cancer treatment showed that low- and moderate-intensity aerobic exercise programs were equally effective in improving physiologic and psychologic function in this population of cancer survivors.[58] Aerobic exercise appeared to be a valuable and well-tolerated component of the cancer rehabilitation process. Patients being treated for colon cancer have decreased quality of life (QOL), mostly due to treatment side effects.[59] There is a positive correlation between improved QOL and engaging in exercise in people with cancer.[57,59] The amount and frequency of physical activity needed to improve QOL has not been fully defined.

The optimal amount of exercise during colon cancer treatment is not yet known. Information from studies on cancer in general demonstrates an increased QOL and reduction of cardiac risk factors with exercise during cancer treatment. The American Cancer Society states that there are insufficient data to conclude a benefit for starting an exercise program in preventing recurrence of cancer during cancer treatment, but they do propose a probable benefit of increased QOL from exercise started or continued during treatment.

Since exercise appears to impact the development of colorectal cancer, can regular exercise improve survival? Two recent studies demonstrate a positive effect of exercise on colon cancer survival and decreasing recurrence. The Melbourne collaborative research study found that regular exercise was associated with a 48 percent reduction in colorectal cancer specific deaths.[60–62] Meyerhardt and colleagues, in another study, demonstrated that 832 patients with stage III colon cancer involved in physical activity had a 47 percent increase in disease-free survival from colorectal cancer.[62] These investigators also studied the impact of exercise upon mortality in a smaller cohort of 573 women.[62] Increasing levels of physical activity after the diagnosis of stages I to III colorectal cancer was found to reduce the risk of colorectal cancer-specific and overall mortality.

In summary, many studies have demonstrated the effects of exercise on both primary and secondary prevention of colon cancer. Men and women who engage in light to moderate levels of exercise on a regular basis will have less than half the risk of the sedentary individuals as far as colon cancer risks. Exercise appears to have a dose-response in the reduction of colon cancer. The benefit is demonstrated with greater than four hours of exercise per week. The type of exercise needed (aerobic, strength training) has not been fully determined. Further studies are needed on the intensity level of exercise needed. The mechanism by which exercise reduces colon cancer risk appears to involve insulin-like growth factor-1 (IGF-1) as well as reduction in prostaglandins. Exercise during and after colon cancer treatment probably benefits overall survival and quality of life. The initiation of exercise during colon cancer treatment is not well studied. There is recent evidence that QOL, cancer-specific mortality, and overall mortality are improved with exercise after colon cancer is diagnosed. Exercise is beneficial to patients for both primary and secondary prevention of colon cancer. Physical activity should be recommended as primary interventions for colorectal cancer prevention. Please see Table 14.3 for the consensus recommendation regarding colorectal cancer prevention.

Gastrointestinal Bleeding

Gastrointestinal (GI) bleeding is generally associated with peptic ulcers, inflammation, and disorders of low blood flow to the digestive tract. GI bleeding can be obvious (bloody or tarry stools) or be hidden and only become detectable by biochemical analysis of the stool. Marathon runners appear to be at higher risk for GI bleeding. Reports have estimated that there may be as much as 25 percent of scant amounts of occult bleeding in marathon runners.[63,64] Since blood is shunted to the muscles and skin, there can be up

Table 14.3
Consensus Public Health Recommendations on Physical Activity and Colon Cancer Risk

Physical activity recommendation should be included in primary intervention for cancer prevention.
All messages for physical activity should be in the context of reducing the risk of colon cancer rather then preventing cancer.
Physical activity should comprise at least 30–45 minutes of moderate to vigorous activity on most days of the week.
Physical activity should be encouraged at all ages.

Source: Reprinted from *Clinical Gastroenterology and Hepatology*, Volume 1, issue 5, Bi and Triadafilopoulos, "Exercise and gastrointestinal function and disease: An evidence-based review of risks and benefits, p. 11, © 2003, with permission from Elsevier.

to 70 percent decreased blood flow to the intestinal tract in prolonged high intensity physical exertion. This low blood flow state in the intestinal tract can cause injury to the tissues leading to bleeding. Although vigorous exercise may induce some level of mild bleeding in the intestinal tract, for those of us who exercise in a less intense regular fashion, there are significant benefits and less risks. In a prospective cohort study of over 8,000 seniors aged 68 years or older with three years of follow-up for the occurrence of severe gastrointestinal bleeding revealed that regular exercise including walking, gardening, or vigorous physical activity was associated with a significantly decreased risk of bleeding.[64] Also, physical activity has been associated inversely with the risk of diverticular disease in over 47,000 men over four years of follow-up even after controlling for confounding factors such as age, dietary fiber, and fat intake.[65]

Liver Disease

In review of the literature to date, it appears that regular exercise does not have an adverse effect on liver functions. Even patients with acute or chronic hepatitis can tolerate exercise and training within their physical limit. Patients with hepatitis who follow an exercise program have a reduced rehabilitation period, shortened hospital stay, and resume normal activities earlier than those who do not exercise.[66] Patients before orthotopic liver transplantation usually show a reduced physical performance status, which impacts on their daily life and social participation.[67] Liver transplantation recipients reported an improved quality of life when engaging in regular physical activity.[68] Nonalcoholic fatty liver disease (NAFLD) occurs across all age groups and ethnicities and is recognized to occur in 14–30 percent of the general population.[69,70] Primary NAFLD is related to insulin resistance and thus frequently occurs as part of the metabolic changes that accompany obesity, diabetes, and hyperlipidemia. The pathogenesis of steatosis (deposition of fat in the liver) and cellular

Table 14.4
Common Perceptions of the Exercise Effect on GI Disorders with Consensus Statement

Common Perceptions	Level of Scientific Evidence	Consensus Statement
Exercise delays gastric emptying and digestion	Contradictory	Light exercise accelerates gastric emptying; vigorous exercise delays emptying of solids and liquids after the work intensity exceeds 70% Vo_2 max
Exercise accelerates intestinal motility	Contradictory	Exercise has no effect on gastrointestinal motility when diet is carefully controlled
Exercise can relieve chronic constipation	Insufficient	Single study found that exercise has no effect on chronic constipation
Exercise can reduce the risk of colon cancer	Convincing	There is overwhelming epidemiologic evidence that exercise has a protective effect against colon cancer
Exercise can induce gastroesophageal reflux	Convincing	Exercise can induce more frequent and longer reflux episodes, but there is no evidence that this is symptomatic or pathologic
Exercise-induced reflux must be considered in patients with exertion-related chest pain	Probable	Cardiac causes must first be ruled out, and twenty-four–hour pH monitoring is useful
Strenuous exercise can cause GI bleeding	Probable	Athletes performing prolonged, exhaustive exercise are especially susceptible to gastrointestinal bleeding

injury is thought to be related mostly to insulin resistance and oxidative stress. Therefore, management entails identification and treatment of metabolic risk factors, improving insulin sensitivity, and increasing antioxidant defenses in the liver. Moderate amounts of weight loss as well as exercise are associated with improvement in insulin sensitivity and thus are logical treatment modalities for patients with NAFLD who are overweight or obese.[71,72] Trials

Table 14.5
Summary of the Most Important Benefits and Risks (If Any) of Exercise on Gastrointestinal Organs

	Benefits	Risks
Esophagus	None	Exacerbation of acid reflux
Stomach	Light exercise accelerates emptying of stomach contents	Emptying of food and inhibits gastric acid production
Small intestine	None	Vigorous exercise may interfere with absorption and promote bleeding
Colon	Reduction of colon cancer risk and risk for diverticular disease	Vigorous exercise may promote bleeding
Liver	May improve fatty liver disease	Probably none

Gastrointestinal Concerns in Various People	Problems	Solutions
Marathoners	A lot of problems with unwanted pit stops, abdominal cramps, and diarrhea	Reduce your intake of high fiber cereals. You don't need the roughage! Fiber increases fecal bulk and movement, thereby reducing transit time. Triathletes with a high fiber intake reported more GI complaints than those with a lower fiber intake. Limit "sugar-free" foods such as sugar-free gum and hard candies.
Runner's Trots	"Jostling" of the intestines; reduced blood flow to the intestines as the body diverts blood; flow to the working muscles; changes in intestinal hormones; altered absorption; dehydration	Exercise lightly before the event to help empty the bowels, drink extra water to maintain hydration.
Dieters	More likely than non-dieters to report abdominal pain, bloating, diarrhea and constipation	

(continued)

Table 14.5
(*continued*)

Gastrointestinal Concerns in Various People	Problems	Solutions
Prior to an interview	In a random survey of 2,500 Americans, 40% reported some form of problem: abdominal pain (22%), bloating (16%), diarrhea (27%). These problems were more prevalent than expected and more prevalent among women than men.	

Source: www.nancyclarkrd.com.

Table 14.6
Definitions of Some Terms Used in the Chapter

Diagnosis	Definition
Peptic Ulcer Disease	A disease characterized by ulcers or breaks in the inner lining (mucosa) of the stomach or duodenum (region of the small intestine closest to the stomach). The three major causes of peptic ulcer disease are non-steroidal anti-inflammatory drugs (NSAIDS), chronic Heliobacter pylori infection, and states of acid hypersecretion, like Zollinger-Ellison syndrome.
Crohn's Disease	A chronic inflammatory disease of the digestive tract, especially involving the small intestine and large intestine
Colitis	Inflammation of the lining of the large intestine

examining the effect of diet and exercise have shown benefit by reductions in liver chemistries that are thought to be elevated from liver inflammation and damage.[73–76] NAFLD is now acknowledged to be the commonest liver condition in the Western world, largely because of the considerable increase in metabolic diseases such as obesity and diabetes. It is clear that NAFLD leads to liver related morbidity and mortality in a subset of people, particularly those who are obese, diabetic, and who have hepatic inflammation. Exercise and diet remain the cornerstone of therapy.

CONCLUSIONS

In general, light to moderate exercise is well tolerated and can benefit patients with various forms of gastrointestinal disease. If there is a significant problem with GERD, avoiding high agitation levels would be beneficial. Otherwise, light to moderate physical activity can benefit gastric emptying, decrease gastric acid production, improve constipation, and help the quality of life of those with inflammatory bowel disease. There is an overwhelming body of evidence to support the role of exercise in preventing development of colon cancer. Even in patients with various forms of liver disease, there is no need for limitation in exercise and actually in the population with NAFLD, exercise is a key component of improving their underlying liver disease. Severe strenuous exercise can have harmful consequences on your digestive health. Exhaustive exercise can interfere with the absorption and assimilation of nutrients and cause gastrointestinal bleeding. Light to moderate exercise should be part of one's health maintenance program.

REFERENCES

1. Keeffe EB, Lowe DK, Goss JR, Wayne R. "Gastrointestinal symptoms of marathon runners." *West J Med* 141 (1984): 481–484.

2. Sullivan SN, Wong C. "Does running cause gastrointestinal symptoms? A survey of 93 randomly selected runners compared with controls." *N Z Med J* 107 (1994): 328–330.

3. Yazaki E, Shawdon A, Beasley I, Evans DF. "The effects of different types of exercise on gastro-oesophageal reflux." *Aust J Sci Med Sort* 28 (1996): 93–96.

4. Clark CS, Kraus BB, Sinclair J, Castell DO. "Gastroesophageal reflux induced by exercise in healthy volunteers." *JAMA* 261 (1989): 3599–3601.

5. Kraus BB, Sinclari JW, Castell DO. "Gastroesophgeal reflux in runners. Characteristics and treatment." *Ann Intern Med* 112 (1990): 429–433.

6. Peters HP, De Kort AF, Van Drevelen H, Akkermans LM, Van Berge Henegouwen GP, Bol E. "The effect of omeprazol on gastro-eosophageal reflux and symptoms during strenuous exercise." *Aliment Pharmacol Ther* 13 (1999): 1015–1022.

7. Cordain L, Latin RW, Behnke JJ. "The effects of an aerobic running program on bowel transit time." *J Sports Med* 26 (1986): 101–104.

8. Cammack J, Read NW, Cann PA, Greenwood B, Holgate AM. "Effect of prolonged exercise on the passage of a solid meal through the stomach and small intestine." *Gut* 23 (1982): 957–961.

9. Cheng Y, Macera CA, Davis Dr, Blari SN. "Physical activity and peptic ulcer. Does physical activity reduce the risk of developing peptic ulcer?" *West J Med* 173 (2000): 101–107.

10. Katshinski BD, Logan RF, Edmond M, Langman MJ. "Physical activity at work and duodenal ulcer risk." *Gut* 32 (1991): 983–986.

11. Sonnenberg A, Hass J. "Joint effect of occupation and nationality on the prevalence of peptic ulcer in German workers." *Br J Ind Med* 43 (1986): 490–493.

12. Sonnenberg A. "Occupational distribution of inflammatory bowel disease among German employees." *Gut* 31 (1990): 1037–1040.

13. Persson PG, Leijonmarck CE, Bernall O, Hellers G, Ahlbom A. "Risk indicators for inflammatory bowel disease." *Int J Epidemiol* 22 (1993): 268–272.

14. Ahlstrøm O, Skrede A, Vhile SG Hove H. "Effect of exercise on nutrient digestibility in trained hunting dogs fed a fixed amount of food." *J Nutr* 136 (2006): 2066S–2068S.

15. D'Inca R, Varnier M, Mestriner C, Marines D, D'Odorico A, Sturniolo GC. "Effect of moderate exercise on Crohn's disease patients in remission." *Ital J Gastroenterol Hepatol* 31 (1999): 205–210.

16. Loudon CP, Coroll V, Butcher J, Pawsthorne P, Bernstein CN. "The effects of physical exercise on patients with Crohn's disease." *Am J Gastroenterol* 94 (1999): 697–703.

17. Pedersen BK, Åkerström TA, Nielsen AR, Fischer CP. "Role of myokines in exercise and metabolism." *J Appl Physiol* 103(3) (Sep 2007): 1093–1098.

18. Starkie R, Ostrowski SR, Jauffred S, Febbraio M, Pedersen BK. "Exercise and IL-6 infusion inhibit endotoxin-induced TNF-alpha production in humans." *FASEB J* 17 (2003): 884–886.

19. Kramer HF, Goodyear LJ. "Exercise, MAPK, and NF-{kappa}B signaling in skeletal muscle." *J Appl Physiol* Feb 15, 2007 {Epub ahead of print}.

20. Febbraio MA. "Exercise and inflammation." *J Appl Physiol* Apr 19, 2007 {Epub ahead of print}

21. Jahnsen J, Falch JA, Aadland E, Moweincket P. "Bone mineral density is reduced in patients with Crohn's disease but not in patients with ulcerative colitis: a population based study." *Gut* 40 (1997): 313–319.

22. Bernstein CN, Blanchard JF, Leslie W, Wajda A, Yu BN. "The incidence of fracture among patients with inflammatory bowel disease. A population-based cohort study." *Ann Intern Med* 133 (2000): 795–799.

23. Kondo T, Naruse S, Hayakawa T, Shibata T. "Effect of exercise on gastro duodenal functions in untrained dogs." *Int J Sports Med* 15 (1994): 186–191.

24. De Wever I, Eeckhout C, Vantrappen G, Hellemans J. "Disruptive effect of test meals on interdigestive motor complex in dogs." *Am J Physiol* 235 (1978): E661–E665.

25. Tasler J, Obtulowicz W, Cieszkowski M, Konturek S. "Gastrointestinal secretory function during physical exercise." *Acta Physiol Pol* 25 (1974): 215–226.

26. Haenszel W, Locke FB, Segi M. "A case-controlled study of large bowel cancer in Japan." *J Natl Cancer Inst* 64 (1980): 17–22.

27. Whittmore AS, Wu-Williams AH, Lee M, Shu Z, Gallegher RP, Deng J, et al. "Diet, physical activity, and colorectal cancer among Chinese in North America and China." *J Natl Cancer Inst* 82 (1990): 915–926.

28. Le Marchand L, Wilkens LR, Kolonel LN, Hankin JH, Lyu LC. "Association of sedentary lifestyle, obesity, smoking, alcohol use, and diabetes with the risk of colorectal cancer." *Cancer Res* 57 (1997): 4787–4794.

29. Wu AH, Paganini-Hill A, Ross RK, Henderson BE. "Alcohol, physical activity and other risk factors for colorectal cancer: a prospective study." *Br J Cancer* 55 (1987): 687–694.

30. Ballard BR, Schatzkin A, Albanes D, Schiffman MH, Kreger BE, Kannel WB, et al. "Physical activity and risk of large bowel cancer in the Framingham Study." *Cancer Res* 50 (1990): 3610–3613.

31. Lee IM, Paffenbarger RS, Hsieh CC. "Physical activity and risk of developing colorectal cancer among college alumni." *J Natl Cancer Inst* 83 (1991): 1324–1329.

32. Giovannucci E, Ashcerio A, Rimm EB, Colditz GA, Stampfer MJ, Willett WC. "Physical activity, obesity, and risk for colon cancer and adenoma in men." *Ann Intern Med* 122 (1994): 327–334.

33. Severson RK, Nomura AM, Gover JS, Stemmenermann GN. "A prospective analysis of physical activity and cancer." *Am J Epidemiol* 130 (1989): 522–529.

34. Gerhardsson M, Norell SE, Kviranta H, Pedersen NL, Ahlbom A. "Sedentary jobs and colon cancer." *Am J Epidemiol* 123 (1986): 775–780.

35. Fraser G, Pearce N. "Occupational physical activity and risk of cancer of the colon, and rectum in New Zealand males." *Cancer Cases Control* 4 (1993): 45–50.

36. Little J, Logan RF, Hawtin PG, Hardcastel JD, Turner ID. "Colorectal adenomas and energy intake, body size and physical activity: A case-controlled study of subjects participating in the Nottingham faecal occult blood screening programme." *Br J Cancer* 67 (1993): 172–176.

37. Tang R, Want JY, Lo SK, Hsieh LL. "Physical activity, water intake and risk of colorectal cancer in Taiwan: A hospital-based case-control study." *Int J Cancer* 82 (1999): 484–489.

38. Kato I, Tominaga S, Matsuura A, Yoshii Y, Shirai M, Kobayashi S. "A comparative case-control study of colorectal cancer and adenoma." *Jpn J Cancer Res* 81 (1990): 1101–1108.

39. Garabrant DH, Peters JM, Mack TM, Bernstein L. "Job activity and colon cancer risk." *Am J Epidemiol* 119 (1984): 1005–1014.

40. Vena JE, Graham SZ, Zielezny M, Swanson MK, Barnes RE, Nolan J. "Lifetime occupational exercise and colon cancer." *Am J Epidemiol* 123 (1985): 775–780.

41. Shephard RJ, Futcher R. "Physical activity and cancer: How may protection be maximized?" *Crit Rev Oncog* 8 (1997): 219–272.

42. Martinez ME, et al. "Leisure-time physical activity, body size, and colon cancer in women. Nurses' Health Study Research Group." *J Natl Cancer Inst* 89 (1997): 948–955.

43. Van Nieuwenhoven MA, F. Brouns, R.M. Brummer. "The effect of physical exercise on parameters of gastrointestinal function." *Neurogastroenterol Motil* 11 (1999): 431–439.

44. Bingham SA, Cummings JH. "Effect of exercise and physical fitness on large intestinal function." *Gastroenterology* 97 (1989): 1389–1399.

45. Soffer EE, Summers RW, Gisolfi C. "Effect of exercise on intestinal motility and transit in trained athletes." *Am J Physiol* 260 (1991): G698–G702.

46. Meshkinpour H, Kemp C, Fairshter R. "Effect of aerobic exercise on mouth-to-cecum transit time." *Gastroenterology* 96 (1989): 938–941.

47. Simon HB. "The immunology of exercise: a brief review." *JAMA* 252 (1984): 2735–2738.

48. Koenuma M, Yamori T, Tsuruo T. "Insulin and insulin-like growth factor 1 stimulate proliferation of metastatic variants of colon carcinoma 26." *Jpn J Cancer Res* 80 (1989): 51–58.

49. Watkins LF, Lewis LR, Levine AE. "Characterization of the synergistic effects of insulin and transferring and the regulation of their receptors on a human colon carcinoma cell line." *Int J Cancer* 45 (1990): 372–375.

50. Williams JC, Walsh DA, Jackson JF. "Colon carcinoma and diabetes mellitus." *Cancer* 54 (1984): 3070–3071.

51. Steenland K, Nowlin S, Palu S. "Cancer incidence in the National Health and Nutrition Survey I follow-up data: Diabetes, cholesterol, pulse, and physical activity." *Cancer Epidemiol Biomarkers Prev* 4 (1995): 807–811.

52. Giovannucci E, Rimm EB, Stampfer MJ, Colditz GA, Asherio A, Willet WC, Speizer FE. "Aspiring and the risk of colorectal cancer and adenoma in male health professionals." *Ann Intern Med* 121 (1994): 241–246.

53. Giovannucci E, Egan KM, Hunter DJ, Stampfer MJ, Colditz GA, Willett WC, Speizer FE. "Aspirin and the risk of colorectal cancer in women." *N Engl J Med* 333 (1994): 609–614.

54. Cruz-Correa M, Shoskes DA, Sanchez P, et al. "Combination treatment with curcumin and quercetin of adenomas in familial adenomatous polyposis." *Clin Gastroenterol Hepatol* 4 (2006): 1035–1038.

55. McTiernan A. "Physical activity after cancer: Physiologic outcomes." *Cancer Invest* 22 (2004): 68–81.

56. Mustian KM, et al. "Exercise and side effects among 749 patients during and after treatment for cancer: a University of Rochester Cancer Center Community Clinical Oncology Program Study." *Support Care Cancer* 14 (2006): 732–741.

57. Burnham TR. "Effects of exercise on physiological and psychological variables in cancer survivors." *Med Sci Sports Exerc* 34 (2002): 1863–1867.

58. Andersen C, et al. "The effect of a multidimensional exercise program on symptoms and side-effects in cancer patients undergoing chemotherapy—the use of semi-structured diaries." *Eur J Oncol Nurs* 10 (2006): 247–262.

59. Haydon AM, et al. "Physical activity, insulin-like growth factor 1, insulin-like growth factor binding protein 3, and survival from colorectal cancer." *Gut* 55 (2006): 689–694.

60. Meyerhardt JA, et al. "Impact of physical activity on cancer recurrence and survival in patients with stage III colon cancer: findings from CALGB 89803." *J Clin Oncol* 24 (2006): 3535–3541.

61. Meyerhardt JA, et al. "Physical activity and survival after colorectal cancer diagnosis." *J Clin Oncol* 24 (2006): 3527–3534.

62. McMahon LF, Ryan MJ, Larson D, Fisher RL. "Occult gastrointestinal blood loss in marathon runners." *Ann Intern Med* 100 (1984): 846–847.

63. Stewart JG, Ahlquist DA, McGill DB, Listrup DM, Schwartz S, Owen RA. "Gastrointestinal blood loss and anemia in runners." *Ann Intern Med* 100 (1984): 843–845.

64. Scobie BA. "Gastrointestinal emergencies with marathon type running: Omental infarction with pancreatitis and liver failure with portal vein thrombosis." *N Z Med J* 111 (1998): 208–210.

65. Aldoori WH, Giovanuucci EL, Rimm EB, Asherio A, Stampfer MJ, Colditz GA, et al. "Prospective study of physical activity and the risk of symptomatic diverticular disease in men." *Gut* 36 (1994): 276–282.

66. Ishida A, Sumiya N, Ueno F. "The effects of physical activity on rehabilitation for acute hepatitis." *Tokai J Exp Clin Med* 21 (1996): 1–6.

67. Painter P, Kransnoff J, Paul SM, Asher NL. "Physical activity and health-related quality of life in liver transplant recipients." *Liver Transplant* 7 (2001): 213–219.

68. Browning J, Szczepaniak L, Dobbins R, et al. "Prevalence of hepatic steatosis in an urban population in the United States: impact of ethnicity." *Hepatology* 40 (2004): 1387–1395.

69. Nomura H, Kashiwagi S, Hayashi J, et al. "Prevalence of fatty liver in a general population of Okinawa, Japan." *Jpn J Med* 27 (1988): 142–149.

70. Petersen KF, Dufour S, Befroy D, et al. "Reversal of nonalcoholic hepatic steatosis, hepatic insulin resistance, and hyperglycemia by moderate weight reduction in patients with type 2 diabetes." *Diabetes* 54 (2005): 603–608.

71. Houmard JA, Tanner CJ, Slentz CA, et al. "Effect of the volume and intensity of exercise training on insulin sensitivity." *J Appl Physiol* 96 (2004): 101–106.

72. Andersen T, Gluud C, Franzmann MB, et al. "Hepatic effects of dietary weight loss in morbidly obese subjects." *J Hepatol* 12 (1991): 224–229.

73. Huang MA, Greenson JK, Chao C, et al. "One-year intense nutritional counseling results in histological improvement in patients with non-alcoholic steatohepatitis: a pilot study." *Am J Gastroenterol* 100 (2005): 1072–1081.

74. Okita M, Hayashi M, Sasagawa T, et al. "Effect of a moderately energy-restricted diet on obese patients with fatty liver." *Nutrition* 17 (2001): 542–547.

75. Palmer M, Schaffner F. "Effect of weight reduction on hepatic abnormalities in overweight patients." *Gastroenterology* 99 (1990): 1408–1413.

76. Ueno T, Sugawara H, Sujaku K, et al. "Therapeutic effects of restricted diet and exercise in obese patients with fatty liver." *J Hepatol* 27 (1997): 103–107.

INDEX

About the Editors and Contributors

Editors

JULIE K. SILVER, M.D., is Assistant Professor, Harvard Medical School, Department of Physical Medicine and Rehabilitation, and is on the medical staff at Dana Farber Cancer Institute, Brigham & Women's, Massachusetts General and Spaulding Rehabilitation Hospitals—all Harvard teaching institutions—in Boston, Massachusetts. Silver has authored, edited, or coedited more than a dozen books including the medical textbook *Clinical Sports Medicine: Medical Management and Rehabilitation* and the consumer trade books *Super Healing* and *After Cancer Treatment: Heal Faster, Better, Stronger.* Silver also coedited Praeger's *Polio Voices: An Oral History from the American Polio Epidemics and Worldwide Eradication Efforts.* She is also Series Editor for two Praeger series, Contemporary Health and Wellness, and Rehabilitation and Recovery after Injury or Disease. Silver has won many awards for her writing and her work has been featured on The Today Show, The Early Show, ABC News Now, NPR and AARP Radio. For more information, visit her Web site at www.juliesilvermd.com.

CHRISTOPHER MORIN, M.S., M.Ed., received a degree in biology from the College of the Holy Cross in 1987, where he was a Hiatt scholar and member of the football and track teams. Morin has also competed in and won many body-building titles without the use of any drugs. He received his first advanced degree from the University of Massachusetts at Amherst in Exercise Science. In order to develop a more varied background for his personal training business, he received a second Master's degree in Health and Fitness from Springfield College. Morin has been in the fitness industry for more than two decades and is an expert in exercise instruction and sports nutrition. He owns FitTec in Massachusetts and is the founder of the American Fitness Testing Association (AFTA, which is dedicated to increasing exercise adherence and motivation). For more information, visit his Web site at www.fiteval.com.

CONTRIBUTORS

DIANE G. ADAMS is a research associate and patient advocate for fibromyalgia at Oregon Health and Science University.

BRENT ALVAR, Ph.D., C.S.C.S.*D, is an assistant research professor in exercise and wellness at Arizona State University.

GHAZALEH ARAM, M.D., is a postdoctoral fellow in gastroenterology and hepatology at Johns Hopkins University.

JENNIFER BAIMA, M.D., is a clinical instructor in physical medicine and rehabilitation at Harvard Medical School.

MATTHEW N. BARTELS, M.D., M.P.H., is the John A. Downey Associate Professor of Clinical Rehabilitation Medicine at the Columbia College of Physicians and Surgeons.

GEORGE L. BLACKBURN, M.D., Ph.D., is the S. Daniel Abraham Associate Professor of Nutrition at Harvard Medical School.

PHILIP BLOUNT, M.D., is an assistant professor of medicine at the University of Mississippi Medical Center.

DANIEL DODD, M.S., C.S.C.S., is a doctoral candidate in physical activity, nutrition, and wellness at Arizona State University.

JASON E. FRANKEL, M.D., is a clinical instructor at Tufts New England Medical Center, Department of Physical Medicine and Rehabilitation.

OSAMA HAMDY, M.D., Ph.D., FACE, is the Medical Director of the Obesity Clinical Program at Joslin Diabetes Center, Harvard University.

NICHOLAS S. HILL, M.D., is Chief of Pulmonary, Critical Care and Sleep Medicine at Tufts-New England Medical Center and Professor of Medicine at Tufts University School of Medicine.

JANICE H. HOFFMAN, B.A., is a clinical exercise specialist with the American Council on Exercise.

JEFFREY C. IVES, Ph.D., is Associate Professor and Graduate Program Chair of Exercise Science at Ithaca College.

KIM DUPREE JONES, Ph.D., is Associate Professor of Nursing and Medicine at Oregon Health and Science University.

WILLIAM MOSI JONES, M.D., is an attending physician at Andrews Institute for Orthopaedics and Sports Medicine.

BETSY KELLER, Ph.D., is a professor of exercise and sport sciences at Ithaca College.

JENNIFER MORIN, M.S., owns FitTec Personal Training of Massachusetts with Christopher Morin.

GERARD MULLIN, M.D., M.H.S., is Director of Integrative GI Nutrition Services at Johns Hopkins University.

DANIEL S. ROOKS, Sc.D., FACSM, is Associate Director of Musculoskeletal Diseases in Translational Medicine at Novartis Institutes for BioMedical Research.

JACQUELINE SHAHAR, M.Ed., R.C.E.P., C.D.E., is a manager in the Exercise Physiology Department and a certified diabetes educator and clinical exercise physiologist at the Joslin Diabetes Center.

JAMES WHORTON is Professor of the History of Medicine at University of Washington School of Medicine.

KATHLEEN Y. WOLIN, Sc.D., is Assistant Professor, Department of Surgery, Washington University School of Medicine.